Get Through
MRCOG Part 2: EMQs

This book is dedicated to Theresia Kien Konje and Augustine Konje Tabe, my parents, for the sacrifice they made to make my dreams come true.

Get Through
MRCOG Part 2: EMQs

Justin C Konje MD FWACS FMCOG(Nig) FRCOG
Professor of Obstetric and Gynaecology and MRCOG Part 2 Course Director,
University of Leicester, Leicester, UK

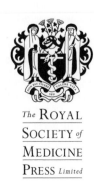

The ROYAL
SOCIETY *of*
MEDICINE
PRESS *Limited*

© 2010 Royal Society of Medicine Press Ltd

Published by the Royal Society of Medicine Press Ltd
1 Wimpole Street, London W1G 0AE, UK
Tel: +44 (0)20 7290 2921
Fax: +44 (0)20 7290 2929
Email: publishing@rsm.ac.uk
Website: www.rsmpress.co.uk

British Library Cataloguing in Publication Data
A catalogue record for this book is available from the British Library

ISBN: 978-1-85315-847-6

Distribution in Europe and Rest of the World:
Marston Book Services Ltd
PO Box 269
Abingdon
Oxon OX14 4YN, UK
Tel: +44 (0)1235 465500
Fax: +44 (0)1235 465555
Email: direct.order@marston.co.uk

Distribution in the USA and Canada:
Royal Society of Medicine Press Ltd
c/o BookMasters Inc
30 Amberwood Parkway
Ashland, OH 44805, USA
Tel: +1 800 247 6553/+1 800 266 5564
Fax: +1 419 281 6883
Email: order@bookmasters.com

Distribution in Australia and New Zealand:
Elsevier Australia
30–52 Smidmore Street
Marrickville NSW 2204, Australia
Tel: +61 2 9517 8999
Fax: +61 2 9517 2249
Email: service@elsevier.com.au

Typeset by Techset Composition Limited, Salisbury, UK
Printed and bound in Great Britain by Bell & Bain, Glasgow

Contents

Preface

Running a successful MRCOG Part 2 revision course has been one of the most satisfying adventures I have ever embarked upon. I have, through the years, provided tuition and support for many new members and fellows of the RCOG who are currently practising in different parts of the world. These courses have been both challenging and educational, as I continue to evolve them. This book is a culmination of this educational process. It is based on where I see deficiencies in candidates and on my own personal experiences regarding the standards of the MRCOG Part 2 examination.

I hope that the contents of this book will spur candidates to work harder and achieve success in their examinations.

I would like to thank my family, Monique, Justin Jr and Swiri, and especially my wife, Joan Kila, for putting up with me while I spend endless hours away from the children running the courses and, more particularly, while I was writing this book.

JK

Introduction

Extended matching questions (EMQs) were introduced into the MRCOG Part 2 examination in September 2006. Their introduction has significantly improved the validity of the MRCOG examination, increased the scope with which various aspects of the curriculum can be assessed and improved the ability of examiners to more objectively assess the clinical competence of trainees. EMQs are widely used for most undergraduate examinations and it is therefore envisaged that candidates will be familiar with this type of examination. The EMQ part of the examination encourages deductive reasoning rather than testing the candidates' ability to memorize facts and recall them when challenged.

The MRCOG Part 2 EMQ paper consists of 40 questions often grouped under various themes, which are virtual (i.e. these are not obvious to the candidate during the examination but the examiner would have set the question based on this theme). The paper is of 1 hour's duration. It contributes 15% of the overall written marks for the examination and there is no negative marking, i.e. no marks are deducted for incorrect answers. Candidates should remember that the written examination is a complete examination and, while it is not necessary to pass all three parts to qualify for progression to the oral part, it is highly desirable to do well in all of the sections.

Preparing for the MRCOG Part 2 examination

The best preparation for the MRCOG Part 2 examination is to use a good teacher – and that is the patient. It is a clinical examination and you cannot substitute theory for experience. Admittedly, your theoretical knowledge should be of a high standard for you to be able to gain from clinical exposure.

Where do you seek this theoretical knowledge? The first source is the RCOG education material. This ought to be the main source of your knowledge. There are several publications by the RCOG which contain the most up-to-date evidence-based materials for your revision. These include:

Green-top Guidelines
The Obstetrician & Gynaecologist
A Guide to the Part 2 MRCOG
MRCOG and Beyond series
www.stratog.net

Other essential reading materials include:

CEMACH reports, available at www.cemach.org.uk: anyone preparing for the examination should read the latest report. It is the most important audit of obstetrics in the UK and it drives the practice of obstetrics until each new report is produced.
NICE guidelines, available at www.nice.org.uk: these are used not only by hospitals but by the RCOG. Candidates should not forget that these guidelines are produced by members and fellows of the RCOG.

Scottish Intercollegiate Network Guidelines (SIGN), available at www.sign.ac.uk: these guidelines are as informative and up to date as the NICE guidelines.

It is my view that you should have one standard textbook in gynaecology and one in obstetrics. Since the examination is about UK practice, the books should be edited by UK clinicians or should have a significant input from UK practitioners. The textbook of choice should not be too superficial but should be detailed enough to include aspects of basic sciences where applicable. It has been my practice to recommend:

Shaw RW, Soutter WP, Stanton SL (eds). *Gynaecology*, 3rd edn. London: Churchill Livingstone, 2002

James DK, Steer PJ, Weiner CP, Gonik B. *High Risk Pregnancy*, 3rd edn. London: Saunders, 2005

Edmonds K. *Dewhurst's Textbook of Obstetrics and Gynaecology*, 7th edn. London: Wiley-Blackwell, 2007. [Remains the standard combined textbook for postgraduates but it makes several assumptions and, therefore, if you are using this as your main textbook, you must also use additional basic textbooks.]

Latest editions of the *Progress in Obstetrics and Gynaecology* series published by Churchill Livingstone and *Recent Advances in Obstetrics and Gynaecology* series, published by the Royal Society of Medicine Press.

Most journals publish review articles and these are areas where you should focus on since they are often reviews of contemporary knowledge of the topics and provide excellent revision materials. The journals you should refer to include:

American Journal of Obstetrics & Gynecology
BJOG: An International Journal of Obstetrics and Gynaecology
BMJ
JAMA, The Journal of the American Medical Association
The Lancet
The New England Journal of Medicine
Obstetrical & Gynecological Survey
Obstetrics and Gynecology

I consider the *Past Papers MRCOG Part Two Multiple Choice Questions, 1997–2001*, published by RCOG Press, to be a must for all candidates. Most of the questions in the book remain valid and should serve as an excellent revision template for candidates.

Since their introduction, there have been many books written on EMQs. As they provide candidates with clues on how to approach papers and the type of questions that can be expected, the books are invaluable guides for the preparation for examinations. However, be careful about the books that you select, as some of the writers have not been fully educated or trained in the best way to generate the questions.

I am also conscious of the fact that there are several websites and 'experts' claiming to have the answers to past multiple choice questions. Candidates are therefore tempted to spend a fortune buying these answers and memorizing them. This is not advisable and, having served on the examination MCQ subcommittee for 6 years, I regard this approach as dangerous and counterproductive.

Finally, make an effort to attend one of the revision courses that are available nationally and internationally. These courses will help you in the preparation for your examinations. If you perform poorly at them, do not be discouraged. On the other hand, do not be complacent if you performed well. Most of the time, they do not reflect your final performance as you will normally continue to work and study after completing the course.

If you have the theoretical knowledge and the clinical experience, you will still need to prepare for the examination in order to understand the techniques that are valuable for answering the questions. You may acquire these skills from courses or through practice and discussions with colleagues.

How to answer EMQs

The most dangerous thing is to start by reading the options list. This will lure you into a false sense of security – and ensure that you get the answer wrong. A good EMQ should have at least three possible correct answers but, when these are then arranged in order of 'which is the most likely', only one will stand out.

Remember that an EMQ consists of four parts – the theme, the options, the instructions, or lead-in-statement, and the items. The theme is 'virtual' but easy to guess from the questions and the list of options. The instructions, or lead-in statement, provide the link between the items and the list of options. It is this section that defines the tasks and enables you to relate the options to the items.

Candidates should, therefore, start by reading this most crucial statement. Once that has been clearly understood, look at the items and note one or two possible answers to each item. If possible, write these on a piece of paper. Go through this process for all the items. Once you have completed the items, go through the list of options looking for your answers. If they are not there, look for the one closest to your answer.

When you do not know the answer, you should be able to make an educated guess. This is more difficult than guessing in other types of MCQs. However, the first thing that you should do is eliminate the incorrect answers. There are likely to be many of them. When guessing, you should remember that common things occur commonly. Always remember that distracters are included in items to ensure that you think clearly about your answer.

How to use this book

Get Through MRCOG Part 2: EMQs is an attempt to make revising for this part of the examination easier. It should be used as an *aide-mémoire* for revising EMQs. It is divided into 8 papers each consisting of 40 questions (i.e. a full examination standard paper). You should use the book as an examination practice template and time yourself as you go through each paper. Answer each paper as if you were sitting an exam and only look at the answers after completing the test. Use the answers to correct and assess your performance. You should then use the explanations to help you understand the reasoning behind some of the answers. There will undoubtedly be questions where you and others disagree with my answers. This is quite a common occurrence with EMQs and I would be surprised if this did not happen many times. When it does happen, please accept that these differences are bound to occur and feel free to make a strong case to yourself and others about the difference of opinion. I hope that this will stimulate discussion around the subject and ultimately enhance understanding.

Option list for Question 1

A.	Coitus interruptus
B.	Condom
C.	Copper multiload intrauterine device
D.	Diaphragm
E.	Fifty (50) μg ethinylestradiol combined oral contraceptive pill
F.	Levonorgestrel intrauterine system (Mirena)
G.	Medroxyprogesterone acetate (Depo-Provera)
H.	Mifepristone
I.	Natural family planning
J.	Progestogen-only oral contraceptive pill
K.	Sequential combined oral contraceptive pill
L.	Sterilization – female
M.	Sterilization – male
N.	Subdermal implant (Implanon or Norplant)
O.	Thirty (30) μg ethinylestradiol combined oral contraceptive pill
P.	Triphasic combined oral contraceptive pill

Instructions: A couple are attending for contraceptive advice. Select the **single** most suitable form of contraception from the option list above.

G 1) A 30-year-old woman had a spontaneous delivery of her fifth child 6 days ago. She is breastfeeding and would like an effective form of contraception as soon as possible. Her body mass index (BMI) is 29 kg/m^2.

Option list for Questions 2–4

A.	Cataract
B.	Caudal regression syndrome
C.	Coarctation of the aorta
D.	Contracture deformities of the limbs
E.	Hypoplastic left ventricle
F.	Hydrops fetalis
G.	Intracranial calcifications
H.	Micrognathia
I.	Phocomelia
J.	Renal agenesis
K.	Scarring of the limbs
L.	Spina bifida
M.	Splenomegaly
N.	Stippled epiphysis
O.	Thrombocytopenia

Instructions: For each of the following infections in pregnancy, select the **single** most likely congenital malformation that it may cause during the first trimester from the option list above. Each option may be selected once, more than once or not at all.

G 2) *Toxoplasma gondii.*

M 3) Cytomegalovirus (CMV).

F 4) Parvovirus B19.

Option list for Questions 5–6

A.	Cimetidine (Tagamet)
B.	Chlopromazine
C.	Chronic renal failure
D.	Empty sella syndrome
E.	Fracture at the base of the skull
F.	Haloperidol
G.	Hypothyroidism
H.	Idiopathic
I.	Lactation
J.	Methyldopa (Aldomet)
K.	Metoclopramide (Maxolon)
L.	Pituitary prolactinoma
M.	Polycystic ovary syndrome (PCOS)
N.	Reserpine (Serpasil)
O.	Stress/anxiety

Instructions: For each of the following case scenarios choose the **single** most likely cause of hyperprolactinaemia from the option list above. Each option may be selected once, more than once or not at all.

5) A 33-year-old woman receiving methyldopa for the treatment of essential hypertension for the past 7 years attends the clinic with secondary amenorrhoea and infertility. On examination, her BMI is 30 kg/m^2. Her hormone profile is as follows: follicle-stimulating hormone (FSH) = 3.5 IU/L, luteinizing hormone (LH) = 8.9 IU/L, free thyroxine (T$_4$) = 12 pmol/L (normal range 9.0–25.0 pmol/L), thyroid-stimulating hormone (TSH) = 2.5 mIU/L (normal range 0.30–5.00 mIU/L), free androgen index = 8.2% (normal 0–6.1%), prolactin = 1025 mIU/L (50–400 mIU/L).

6) A 30-year-old woman presents with inappropriate galactorrhoea and associated loss of libido. On examination, her BMI is 29 kg/m^2. A pelvic ultrasound scan revealed five or six multiple peripheral follicles in each ovary, the maximum diameter of each being 8 mm. Her hormone profile is as follows: FSH = 5.7 IU/L, LH = 9.8 IU/L, free T$_4$ = 11 pmol/L, TSH = 5.7 mIU/L and prolactin = 989 mIU/L.

Option list for Question 7

A.	Abdominal ultrasound scan
B.	Amniotomy (ARM)
C.	Admit to the antenatal ward
D.	Continuous cardiotocograph (CTG) with a fetal scalp electrode
E.	Continuous CTG with transabdominal transducer
F.	Corticosteroids
G.	Doppler of the umbilical artery
H.	Emergency caesarean section
I.	Epidural analgesia
J.	Erythromycin, continuous CTG and deliver
K.	External cephalic version
L.	Fetal blood sampling
M.	Group and cross-match
N.	Intravenous broad-spectrum antibiotics, CTG and deliver
O.	Intravenous cannula
P.	Intravenous dextrose saline
Q.	Intravenous oxytocin
R.	Intravenous Ringer's lactate
S.	Intravenous terbutaline
T.	Maternal pulse
U.	Oxygen by facemask
V.	Prostaglandin pessaries
W.	Pulmonary wedge pressure catheter
X.	Re-examine in 4 hours

Instructions: A patient presents to the labour ward as an emergency. Choose the **single** most appropriate immediate action from the option list above.

7) A 34-year-old woman is admitted at 34 weeks' gestation with a 6-day history of confirmed preterm prelabour rupture of the fetal membranes. In addition, she is pyrexial, has a temperature of 38.4°C and there is fetal tachycardia of 180 bpm. The fetal heart rate is, however, reactive with good baseline variability. On vaginal examination the cervix is closed.

Option list for Questions 8–9

A.	Bilateal salpingoophorectomy
B.	Combined oral contraceptive pill
C.	Danazol
D.	Depo-Provera
E.	Endometrial ablation
F.	Gonadotrophin-releasing hormone (GnRH) agonists
G.	Levonorgestrel intrauterine system (Mirena)
H.	Mefenamic acid
I.	Myomectomy (abdominal)
J.	Norethisterone
K.	Reassurance
L.	Total abdominal hysterectomy
M.	Tranexamic acid
N.	Transcervical laser polypectomy
O.	Uterine artery embolization

Instructions: For each of the following clinical scenarios, choose the **single** best long-lasting treatment from the option list above. Each option may be selected once, more than once or not at all.

8) A 40-year-old obese (BMI = 30 kg/m^2) mother of four presents with heavy periods since undergoing sterilization 4 years earlier. A pelvic examination and ultrasound scans were unremarkable. Various medical treatment options have been unsuccessful.

9) A 34-year-old nulliparous teacher presents with dysmenorrhoea and menorrhagia. She has had two miscarriages and was found to have a large submucous fibroid polyp measuring 8 × 9 cm.

Option list for Questions 10–11

A.	Assisted breech delivery
B.	Bakri balloon
C.	Brace suture
D.	Breech extraction
E.	Caesarean section
F.	Emergency caesarean section
G.	Fetal blood sampling
H.	Internal podalic version and breech extraction
I.	Intramuscular syntometrine
J.	Intravenous ergometrine
K.	Kielland's forceps delivery
L.	Neville–Barnes forceps delivery
M.	Packing of the uterus
N.	Recombinant factor VIIa
O.	Transfusion with fresh whole blood
P.	Ventouse delivery with metal cup
Q.	Ventouse delivery with Silastic cup
R.	Wrigley's forceps

Instructions: For each of the following case scenarios choose the **single** most appropriate management option from the option list above. Each option may be used once, more than once or not at all.

10) A 38-year-old primigravida who conceived twins after the fourth attempt at in vitro fertilization (IVF) was induced at 38 weeks' gestation. She delivered the first twin 45 minutes ago. The membranes of the second twin are intact and the twin is lying longitudinally and presenting cephalic. Syntocinon was started 30 minutes ago and uterine contractions resumed shortly after. A sudden unrecovering bradycardia has developed with some brisk vaginal loss.

11) A 30-year-old primigravida had a spontaneous vaginal delivery 2 hours ago following an uncomplicated labour. She developed severe postpartum haemorrhage and failed to respond to all forms of conservative treatment, including cryoprecipitate and fresh frozen plasma. She is reluctant to have surgery except as a last report.

Option list for Questions 12–14

A.	Bowel preparation
B.	Chest X-ray
C.	Electrocardiogram (ECG)
D.	Endocervical swab for *Chlamydia trachomatis*
E.	Examine under anaesthesia and cystoscopy
F.	Full blood count
G.	Group and save
H.	Haemoglobin electrophoresis
I.	Midstream urine for microscopy and sensitivity
J.	Obtain consent
K.	Pregnancy test
L.	Proctosigmoidoscopy
M.	Thrombophilia screen
N.	Ultrasound scan of the abdomen
O.	Urea and electrolytes

Instructions: For each of the following patients being prepared for surgery, select from the option list above the **single** most relevant unique investigation that you would perform on the patient before surgery. Each investigation may be selected once, more than once or not at all.

12) A 30-year-old African–Caribbean woman with lower abdominal pain, dyspareunia and an irregular vaginal discharge is admitted for a diagnostic laparoscopy.

13) A 34-year-odd woman who had a multi-load copper intrauterine device inserted 3 years previously is attending for laparoscopic sterilization as a day case. Her BMI index is 24 kg/m^2.

14) A 17-year-old girl is attending for a surgical termination at 8 weeks' gestation. She was seen in the clinic very briefly by the nurse counsellor who requested an ultrasound scan in order to confirm the gestational age of the pregnancy prior to the termination.

Option list for Questions 15–16

A.	Admission
B.	Admit for daily CTGs
C.	Ampicillin
D.	Analgesics and antibiotics
E.	Appendicectomy
F.	Biophysical profile
G.	Cephalexin
H.	Cholecystectomy
I.	Erythromycin
J.	Induction of labour
K.	Indometacin
L.	Intravenous fluids
M.	Management in haemodialysis unit (HDU)
N.	Magnesium sulphate
O.	Benzylpenicillin
P.	Steroids
Q.	Surgical excision

Instructions: For each of the following clinical scenarios, choose the **single most appropriate treatment** from the option list above. Each option may be used once, more than once or not at all.

15) A 21-year-old woman presents at 36 weeks' gestation with polyhydramnios and fetal macrosomia. She was diagnosed with gestational diabetes mellitus at 28 weeks' gestation after an oral glucose tolerance test (indication – high BMI). She has been put on a controlled diet and the blood glucose test strips (BM stix) have all been within normal limits. She is not in labour but feels uncomfortable lying on her back.

16) A 24-year-old woman is seen as an emergency at 28 weeks with recurring abdominal pain (mainly on the right upper abdomen). The pain is worse soon after eating. It is associated with nausea and vomiting, but this is not thought to be severe enough to warrant admission. On examination, she is tender in the right hypochondrion and an ultrasound scan reveals the presence of two small gallstones.

Option list for Questions 17–18

A.	Allergic reaction
B.	Aphthous ulcer
C.	Bartholin's abscess
D.	Behçet's disease
E.	Cyclic vulvitis
F.	Dysaesthetic vulvodynia
G.	Episodic vulvitis
H.	Essential vulvodynia
I.	Herpes simplex
J.	Lupus erythematosus
K.	Plasma dermatitis
L.	Pyoderma gangrenosa
M.	Vulval dermatoses
N.	Vulval vestibulitis syndrome

Instructions: For each of the following clinical cases, select the **single** most likely cause of vulval pain from the option list above. Each option may be chosen once, more than once or not at all.

17) A 30-year-old woman presents with severe pain in the vulva, which is predominantly at the entrance to the vagina, of 9 months' duration. It is so painful that she cannot have sexual intercourse. There is no associated vaginal discharge. On examination, there is mild erythema involving the vestibule. Pressing the vestibule with a cotton bud elicits severe pains.

18) A 19-year-old woman presents with severe acute-onset vulval pain, difficulties passing urine and a slight temperature. She is not using any form of contraception. Over the past 4 days she has noticed that her pants had been stained with a brownish discharge. On examination, there are multiple vesicles on the vulva but no other abnormality.

Option list for Questions 19–21

A.	Anaemia
B.	Asthma
C.	Bad news
D.	Diabetes mellitus with complications
E.	Domestic violence
F.	Exhaustion
G.	Fear
H.	Heart failure
I.	Hyperventilation anxiety
J.	Idiopathic
K.	Labour
L.	Mitral valve stenosis
M.	Peripartum cardiomyopathy
N.	Physiological (pregnancy related)
O.	Pleural effusion
P.	Pneumonia
Q.	Pneumothorax
R.	Pulmonary embolism
S.	Pulmonary tuberculosis

Instructions: For each of the following clinical scenarios described below, choose from the option list above the **single** most likely cause of the patient's symptoms. Each option may be used once, more than once or not at all.

19) A 33-year-old woman presents at 33 weeks' gestation with breathlessness and wheezing which is worse at night and after exercise. She has had an exacerbation of these symptoms for the past 2 weeks. On examination, she is clinically stable and there are obvious rhonchi in the chest.

20) A 35-year-old grand multiparous woman presents at 33 weeks' gestation with breathlessness of 1 week's duration. She has five young children and no help at home. In addition, she has to work 20 hours a week. On examination, she is clinically comfortable at rest. There is bilateral pitting oedema and a smooth tongue.

F 21) A 29-year-old teacher and mother of three presents at 36 weeks' gestation with breathlessness of 3 weeks' duration. She looks after her children and has continued to teach. She is planning to take maternity leave at 38 weeks. She is not breathless on exertion and describes fetal movements as normal ('whenever I am able to stop and think'). On examination, her pulse is 90 beats per minute (bpm), blood pressure (BP) 135/88 mmHg and urine examination shows glucose ++. The fundal height is 38 cm and a CTG is normal.

Option list for Questions 22–23

A.	Adrenalectomy
B.	Aromatase inhibitors
C.	Bromocriptine
D.	Combined oral contraceptive pill
E.	Corticosteroids
F.	Cyproterone acetate
G.	Danazol
H.	Estrogens
I.	Finasteride
J.	GnRH agonist
K.	Growth hormones
L.	Medroxyprogesterone acetate
M.	Neurosurgical excision
N.	Ovarian cystectomy
O.	Reassurance
P.	Testicular tumour removal
Q.	Thyroxine

Instructions: For each of the following clinical scenarios described below, select from the option list above the **single** most appropriate first-line treatment. Each option may be selected once, more than once or not at all.

J 22) An 8-year-old girl presents with features of precocious puberty and investigations reveal that she has McCune–Albright syndrome.

23) An 18-year-old girl presenting with precocious puberty is investigated and the following abnormal results were found: raised TSH, low FSH and LH levels, normal estrogen levels and multiple cystic lesions in her bones.

Option list for Questions 24–25

A.	Beta blockers
B.	Carbimazole
C.	Cortisol
D.	Diet modification
E.	Erythromycin
F.	Hormone replacement
G.	Intravenous hydrocortisone
H.	Insulin
I.	Levothyroxine
J.	Metformin
K.	Methyldopa
L.	Phenoxybenzamine and alpha blockers
M.	Propylthiouracil
N.	Radioactive iodine
O.	Spironolactone
P.	Synthetic vasopressin
Q.	Surgery

Instructions: For each of the following clinical scenarios described below, choose from the option list above the **single** most effective first-line treatment. Each option may be selected once, more than once or not at all.

24) A 29-year-old woman presents at 8 weeks' gestation for booking. It is her second pregnancy. Following the delivery of her first baby, she suffered from very severe postpartum haemorrhage and was unable to breastfeed. She tried to become pregnant spontaneously but failed and, following investigations in the hospital, was given some injections after which she became pregnant. She is currently not on any medication. On examination, she has a BP of 135/87 mmHg and a pulse of 88 bpm. There is a trace of protein and nitrites + in her urine. An ultrasound confirms a single pregnancy of appropriate gestation.

D 25) A 33-year-old woman books for antenatal care at 7 weeks' gestation. She has had three miscarriages, all between the gestational ages of 6 and 8 weeks. Her BMI is 34 kg/m². She has been suffering from moderate nausea and occasional vomiting, but is not dehydrated. She is reluctant to be admitted. This was a pregnancy conceived after letrozole (as she had failed to achieve a pregnancy with clomifene citrate). On examination she has a trace of protein in her urine.

Option list for Question 26

A.	Aortic stenosis
B.	Arrhythmias
C.	Cerebral oedema
D.	Drug induced
E.	Fluid overload
F.	Hyperglycaemia
G.	Hyperpyrexia
H.	Hypoglycaemia
I.	Hypertrophic cardiomyopathy
J.	Idiopathic hypotension
K.	Labyrinthitis
L.	Massive haemorrhage
M.	Postural hypotension
N.	Sepsis
O.	Supine hypotension syndrome

Instructions: Choose from the option list above the **single** most likely cause of the dizziness with which the following patient presented.

I 26) A 20-year-old woman presents with breathlessness, chest pain and dizzy spells at 32 weeks' gestation. On examination, her BP is 120/77 mmHg and urinalysis is negative. There is, however, a double apical pulsation (palpable fourth heart sound) and a pansystolic murmur.

Option list for Questions 27–28

A.	Amniotic fluid embolism
B.	Cerebral haemorrhage
C.	Cerebral infarction
D.	Cerebral vein thrombosis
E.	Eclampsia
F.	Hypoglycaemia
G.	Hypocalcaemia
H.	Hyponatraemia
I.	Placental abruption
J.	Postpartum haemorrhage
K.	Pulmonary embolism
L.	Ruptured congenital aneurysm
M.	Ruptured uterus
N.	Seizures
O.	Subarachnoid haemorrhage
P.	Vasovagal attack

Instructions: For each of the following clinical scenarios, choose from the option list above the **single** most likely cause of collapse. Each option may be used once, more than once or not at all.

27) A 38-year-old G2P1 is admitted in spontaneous labour at 40 weeks' gestation. Fetal membranes are intact and the CTG is normal. The cervix is 2 cm dilated on admission. One hour after admission she progresses to full cervical dilatation and, following a spontaneous rupture of the membranes, delivered a male baby weighing 3.5 kg. She then develops profound shock and respiratory distress, and is cyanosed on examination. The uterus is poorly contracted and she is bleeding torrentially.

28) A 42 year old is being induced for postdates at 42 weeks' gestation into her third pregnancy – the previous two were surgical terminations at 12 and 16 weeks' gestation, respectively. She was given two prostaglandin pessaries and after an artificial rupture of membranes (ARM) was commenced on Syntocinon. She progressed normally and became fully dilated. She started pushing and suddenly collapsed with associated bradycardia. The baby was delivered immediately with a forceps and has a cord pH of 7.1, base excess (BE) −8 mmol/L. There is significant bleeding from the vagina and the blood is clotting normally.

Option list for Questions 29–30

A.	Breast cancer
B.	Cancer in children
C.	Chromosome abnormalities
D.	Ectopic pregnancy
E.	Endometrial cancer
F.	Growth discordancy in childhood
G.	Hyperemesis gravidarum
H.	Hypospadias
I.	Laparoscopic visceral injury
J.	Multiple pregnancies
K.	Ovarian carcinoma
L.	Ovarian cysts
M.	Ovarian hyperstimulation syndrome
N.	Preterm labour
O.	Prolonged hospitalization
P.	Psychological distress

Instructions: The complications listed above are related to assisted reproduction treatment techniques (ART). For each of the following cases, select from the option list above the **single** most likely complication from which the patient may be suffering. Each option may be selected once, more than once or not at all.

H 29) A couple were investigated for infertility. The man was found to be oligzoospermic and the women had blocked tubes and irregular ovulation. They were therefore offered intracytoplasmic sperm injection (ICSI) with superovulation. They are anxious about the effects of the procedure on the resulting children.

C 30) Several studies have been undertaken to investigate the effect of ICSI on the offspring. There is evidence that these children have a greater risk of a particular complication compared with those from other types of ART.

Option list for Questions 31–34

A.	Acute fatty liver of pregnancy
B.	Cholecystitis
C.	Drug induced
D.	Intracranial tumour
E.	Haemolysis, elevated liver enzymes and low platelet count (HELLP)
F.	Hydatidiform pregnancy
G.	Hypercalcaemia
H.	Hyperemesis gravidarum
I.	Hyperglycaemia
J.	Gastroenteritis
K.	Metabolic causes
L.	Pre-eclampsia
M.	Physiological
N.	Thyrotoxicosis
O.	Uraemia
P.	Urinary tract infection

Instructions: For each of the following clinical scenarios, choose the **single** most likely cause of vomiting from the option list above. Each option may be used once, more than once or not at all

31) A 22-year-old woman presents with abdominal pains, vomiting and increased frequency of bowel motions at 24 weeks' gestation. Her symptoms began 3 days ago when she visited her parents. On examination, she is well hydrated but has a slight pyrexia (temperature = $37.4°C$), BP = 140/95 mmHg; her abdomen is soft but the uterus is irritable. The fundal height measures 24 cm and the fetal heart can be heard and is normal. Her biochemistry is as follows: urea and electrolytes are Na^+ 136 mmol/L, K^+ 4.8 mmol/L, Cl^- 25 mmol/L, HCO_3^- 23 mmol/L, urea 6.2 mmol/L and haemoglobin (Hb) 15.7 g/dL. Urinalysis demonstrated a trace of protein.

B 32) A 20-year-old woman presents with nausea, vomiting and abdominal pains of 3 days' duration. The nausea tends to be worse after eating. She is 21 weeks pregnant and there have been no complications so far. On examination, her temperature is 38.0°C, BP is 120/69 mmHg and her pulse is 101 bpm. There is a marked tenderness over the right hypochondrion and the flank. There are no other abnormalities. Urinalysis reveals traces of protein, leucocytes and blood. Her white cell count was significantly raised.

C 33) A 20-year-old woman is seen in the antenatal clinic complaining of nausea and vomiting of 3 weeks' duration. She is currently 28 weeks pregnant and was started on iron tablets 3 weeks earlier as her Hb had been low. On examination nothing abnormal was found. Her biochemistry is as follows: urea and electrolytes are Na^+ 137 mmol/L, K^+ 6.8 mmol/L, Cl^- 27 mmol/L, HCO_3^- 24 mmol/L, urea 4.5 mmol/L and Hb 10.0 g/dL.

L 34) A 24-year-old woman presents at 18 weeks' gestation with nausea, vomiting and sudden-onset headaches. She has also noticed that she prefers the dark. On examination, her BP is 150/100 mmHg, pulse 90 bpm and her reflexes are brisk. Urinalysis reveals protein $++++$ and blood $++$. The fundal height is 16 cm and the fetal heart is heard and is normal. Her biochemistry is as follows: urea and electrolytes are Na^+ 128 mmol/L, K^+ 6.3 mmol/L, Cl^- 22 mmol/L, HCO_3^- 19 mmol/L, urea 7.5 mmol/L and Hb 13.7 g/dL.

Option list for Questions 35–38

A.	Asherman's syndrome
B.	Autoimmune dysfunction
C.	Anti-thrombin III deficiency
D.	Antiphospholipid syndrome (APS)
E.	Bacterial vaginosis
F.	Hypoplastic uterus
G.	Hyperhomocysteinaemia
H.	Cervical weakness
I.	Protein C deficiency
J.	Protein S deficiency
K.	Lupus anticoagulant
L.	Protein Z deficiency
M.	Hypothyroidism
N.	Unexplained (idiopathic)
O.	Polycystic ovary syndrome
P.	Uterine fibroids

Instructions: For each of the following case scenarios, choose from the option list above the **single** most likely cause of the recurrent miscarriage. Each option may be selected once, more than once or not at all.

35) A 38-year-old P1+3 presents after her third miscarriage for investigations. The miscarriages were at 10, 9 and 8 weeks, respectively. Her periods are regular but very heavy. Her hormone profile was as follows: prolactin = 578 mIU/L (normal up to 400 mIU/L), LH = 6.4 IU/L, FSH = 6.4 IU/L, TSH = 3.4 mIU/L and free T_4 = 12 pmol/L. An ultrasound of the pelvic organs revealed a normal left ovary and a right ovary with suspicions of PCOS: the uterus was described as enlarged and containing a 4×6 cm submucous fibroid located in the upper part of the uterus.

36) A 32 year old presented to the recurrent miscarriage clinic after her third miscarriage. The miscarriages were all at around 8–10 weeks. On each occasion, she had an ultrasound scan at 6 weeks which showed a viable intrauterine pregnancy. However, on each occasion she bled and a further ultrasound scan at 8 weeks revealed an intrauterine fetal death. A thrombophilia screen has so far been negative. Her hormone profile is normal but the rest of the investigations are awaited.

M 37) A 40-year-old woman presents to the recurrent miscarriage clinic after her fifth miscarriage. All the miscarriages were in the first 10 weeks of pregnancy. She is otherwise healthy, although her case notes show that she has been putting on weight and does not like the winter. Nothing abnormal is found on examination. Her hormone profile was a follows: LH = 4.5 IU/L, FSH = 8.7 IU/L, TSH = 15 mIU/L, free T_4 = 9 IU/L, thyroid peroxidase antibody = 163 (normal <20). Ultrasound scan of the ovaries showed four to five tiny follicles in each ovary.

N 38) A 26-year-old woman presented to the recurrent miscarriage clinic after her third miscarriage. The miscarriages were between 5 and 6 weeks' gestation. She is clinically well and physical examination revealed no abnormality. The karyotype of the products from two of the miscarriages was normal. Her hormone profile and thrombophilia screen were all normal. The results of anticardiolipin antibodies and lupus anticoagulant are awaited.

Option list for Questions 39–40

A.	Abdominal ultrasound scan
B.	ARM
C.	Admit to the antenatal ward
D.	Catheterize the bladder
E.	Continuous cardiotocograph (CTG) with a fetal scalp electrode
F.	Continuous CTG with transabdominal transducer
G.	Doppler of the umbilical artery
H.	Emergency caesarean section and IV antibiotics
I.	Epidural analgesia
J.	External cephalic version
K.	Fetal blood sampling
L.	Group and cross-match
M.	Intravenous antibiotics
N.	Intravenous cannula
O.	Intravenous dextrose saline
P.	Intravenous oxytocin
Q.	Intravenous Ringer's lactate
R.	Intravenous terbutaline
S.	Maternal pulse
T.	Oxygen by facemask
U.	Prostaglandin pessaries
V.	Pulmonary wedge pressure catheter
W.	Re-examine in 4 hours
X.	Turn to left side

Instructions: For each of the following clinical scenarios choose from the option list above the **single** most appropriate immediate action. Each option may be used once, more than once or not at all.

39) A 20-year-old primigravida at 37 weeks' gestation was induced for fetal growth restriction. ARM was performed 10 hours ago and meconium-stained liquor was obtained. Intravenous Syntocinon was commenced immediately after the ARM and an hour later she started contracting regularly and strongly. The cervix was 8 cm at

the last vaginal examination. The fetal heart rate has risen from a baseline of 144 bpm to 162 bpm with reduced variability and occasional early decelerations.

40) A 34-year-old woman is admitted at 34 weeks' gestation with a 6-day history of confirmed prelabour preterm rupture of fetal membranes. In addition, she is pyrexial (temperature 38.4°C) and there is a fetal tachycardia of 180 bpm. The fetal heart rate is, however, reactive with a good baseline variability. The cervix is closed on vaginal examination.

1. Practice Paper 1: Answers

1) G.
Many of the options will be considered suitable forms of contraception for this woman; however, because she is breastfeeding, the combined oral contraceptive pill will be unsuitable. Sterilization immediately postpartum is not ideal and should be performed as an interval procedure. Implanon would be appropriate but she will require counselling and then be referred to the appropriate centre where it can be inserted. It is not routinely offered on postnatal wards. Depo-Provera (medroxyprogesterone acetate) is the best option and can be administered before she is discharged from the ward.

2) G.
Although *Toxoplasma gondii* is a recognized cause of several congenital malformations, from the list of options, intracranial calcifications is the most likely congenital malformation.

3) M.
CMV can cause hydrops fetalis, intracranial calcifications, splenomegaly and thrombocytopenia. Hydrops is unlikely following infection in the first trimester – in fact, symmetrical fetal growth restriction is most likely. Although thrombocytopenia is possible this is often a diagnosis made after delivery unless a fetal blood sample is performed. The correct answer is therefore splenomegaly which can be diagnosed from an ultrasound scan.

4) F.
Hydrops fetalis is the obvious answer from the option list. The other malformations are rarely associated with parvovirus B19 infections.

5) M.
The possible causes of hyperprolactinaemia in this patient include drug induced (methyldopa), stress/anxiety and polycystic ovary syndrome. Her high BMI, raised LH/FSH ratio and raised free androgen index will support the diagnosis of PCOS. Drugs and anxiety/stress are less likely to cause such a raised prolactin level.

6) H.
The three possible causes in this patient include PCOS, stress/anxiety and idiopathic. There is nothing in her history to suggest stress/anxiety and the biochemistry and ultrasound findings are not supportive of PCOS. The most likely cause is therefore idiopathic.

7) N.
This patient probably has chorioamnionitis. She should therefore be managed with a combination of broad-spectrum intravenous antibiotics and delivery. The timing of the delivery and the method of delivery will depend on the state of the fetus. A CTG will provide the necessary information.

8) L.
The two options for this patient include the Mirena contraceptive device and hysterectomy. The Mirena could be considered a medical treatment, in which case it is not very suitable. However, since it is inserted as a minor surgical procedure, it should really be considered non-medical. A hysterectomy is the best long-lasting option since not all women using the Mirena will benefit and, indeed, some will eventually require a hysterectomy.

9) N.
A polypectomy is the best option in this case. Not only is the fibroid too large to be left alone but the patient also presented with dysmenorrhoea and menorrhagia – features most likely to be attributable to the fibroids. A myomectomy can be considered but it is not the best option.

10) H.
This baby needs to be delivered as the placenta is most likely to have abrupted. The option must therefore be one that results in the quickest delivery. Since the first twin has already been delivered, and the membranes of the second twin are intact, an internal podalic version and breech extraction will be the quickest way to deliver the baby. An immediate caesarean section will also be acceptable especially if the person delivering the baby does not have the necessary expertise. This was, however, not the question and an assumption must be made that the expertise was available.

11) N.
The only other option left for this patient is recombinant factor VII. All non-surgical options have failed. This is an expensive option and surgery must follow if it fails.

12) H.
Abnormal haemoglobins could make anaesthesia difficult. It is therefore important to exclude this through Hb electrophoresis. Other investigations would apply to most women undergoing this procedure.

13) K.
A pregnancy test is mandatory for all women in the reproductive age group undergoing any surgical procedure, especially for those undergoing sterilization.

14) D.
One of the complications of a termination of pregnancy is pelvic infection from *C. trachomatis* and *Neisseria gonorrhoeae*. An endocervical swab for *Chlamydia* – the most common cause of post-termination pelvic inflammatory disease – will result in early identification and treatment.

15) P.
This diabetic patient has polyhydramnios which is indicative of poor diabetic control. She is 36 weeks and likely to require delivery soon. At this gestational age, one of the most common neonatal problems will be respiratory distress syndrome. Administering steroids will therefore reduce the risk of this complication occurring and reduce its severity if it did occur.

16) H.
The most likely cause of the pain is a gallstone or gallbladder disorder. The preferred treatment is therefore a cholecystectomy.

17) N.
The features presented are in keeping with a vulval inflammatory or infective condition. The erythema and pain on touching the vestibule with a cotton wool are indicative of vulval vestibulitis.

18) I.
Herpes simplex is the most likely cause of the vulval pain in this patient. Her age, the presenting symptoms and the findings on examination point to this diagnosis.

19) B.
The most likely cause of the symptoms in this patient is asthma. She is unlikely to have heart failure as there is nothing in her history that points to this. Hyperventilation anxiety is unlikely to present in this way, although it must be considered as a differential diagnosis.

20) A.
The differential diagnoses in this case include anaemia, asthma, hyperventilation anxiety, fear, idiopathic and exhaustion. Bilateral oedema is present in over 90% of women at this gestational age and hence it is not an important clinical feature. The smooth tongue is characteristic of iron deficiency anaemia which makes anaemia the most likely cause of her symptoms.

21) F.
The features are similar to those of the patient in question 20. However, her physical activities should make the answer very obvious.

22) J.

The physiological basis of precocious puberty in this condition is the abnormal gonadotrophins. Therefore a GnRH agonist is the best treatment option.

23) Q.

This girl is hypothyroid and is likely to have precocious puberty secondary to juvenile hypothyroidism. The treatment option would be a combination of thyroxine and a GnRH agonist. However, thyroxine on its own will reduce the gonadotrophins and, hopefully, arrest any further development of the secondary sexual characteristics.

24) F.

This patient has Sheehan's syndrome which is characterized by panhypopituitarism. The best treatment option is therefore the replacement of the hormones that are regulated by the anterior pituitary using thyroxine and cortisol. It is likely that she achieved pregnancy following gonadotrophin injections.

25) D.

This question requires the candidates to think beyond the information provided. She presents with nausea and vomiting but these are well tolerated. It is easy to immediately think of offering her treatment for these symptoms. However, on the basis of her BMI and ovulation induction with an aromatase inhibitor, she is likely to have PCOS. The risk of this in pregnancy is gestational diabetes and dietary modification and control are the best treatment option.

26) I.

These symptoms are suggestive of a cardiac pathology. The differential diagnoses should therefore include aortic stenosis, arrhythmias and hypertrophic cardiomyopathy. The features easily exclude aortic stenosis and arrhythmia, and thus hypertrophic cardiomyopathy is the most likely option.

27) A.

The patient presented with post delivery collapse. Several causes are possible. However, in this case, the timing of the onset and the associated respiratory distress, cyanosis and massive haemorrhage make amniotic fluid embolism the most likely cause.

28) M.

The features are classic and it is unlikely that there is any cause other than ruptured uterus.

29) H.

Although chromosomal abnormalities have been widely reported to be associated with ICSI, these Y-chromosomal abnormalities are thought to be minor and not clinically relevant. The only abnormality that has been associated with ICSI to a significant degree is hypospadias.

30) C.
Y-chromosomal abnormalities are most commonly associated with ICSI but do not have long-term clinical relevance.

31) J.
This patient has gastroenteritis although other causes must also be considered. Her temperature, vomiting and frequency of bowel motions all point to this diagnosis. Although her BP is elevated, there is no information about her booking BP and her biochemistry is normal, making HELLP unlikely at this gestation.

32) B.
A positive Murphy sign is diagnostic of cholecystitis. While pre-eclampsia could be a differential diagnosis, the patient's temperature makes it highly unlikely. The urinalysis findings could also make urinary tract infections a differential; however, with a temperature of 38°C and leucocytosis one would have expected more evidence of infection in the urine.

33) C.
The history gives the answer away. Everything else is normal and the only provoking factor in this patient is likely to be the iron tablets. Although these are known to cause constipation and dark stools, nausea and vomiting are recognized side effects.

34) L.
Pre-eclampsia is rare at this gestational age. However, this is the most likely diagnosis. High blood pressure, significant proteinuria and the biochemistry certainly point to it. The gestational age at presentation is unusual, but the smaller than normal uterus will suggest a growth-restricted fetus and this, combined with the presentation, will suggest a karyotypical abnormality which is known to present with features of early pre-eclampsia.

35) P.
Uterine fibroids are common and, in most patients, do not cause problems. However, when they are submucous they may cause a miscarriage, especially when the pregnancy implants over them.

36) D.
Miscarriages occurring after the eighth week of gestation, and after fetal viability has been confirmed on ultrasound scan, will point to the APS even though the thrombophilia screen was negative. Autoimmune dysfunction is a recognized cause, but it is not as common as APS. In addition, APS is part of an autoimmune dysfunction.

37) M.

The age of the patient and the raised thyroid peroxidase antibodies all point to a thyroid dysfunction. This is more likely to be a cause in older women and in this patient the TSH is raised while the free T_4 is low. All of these factors point to hypothyroidism.

38) N.

The miscarriages here all occurred early and are therefore likely to be unrelated to any maternal factors. A subserous fibroid is not normally thought to be associated with miscarriages.

39) K.

A decision needs to be made about whether to perform a caesarean section or allow labour to continue. This decision can be made only after a fetal blood sample. None of the other options will allow for this decision to be made with certainty. An emergency caesarean section would not necessarily be the best option and is not in keeping with the recommendations made in the NICE guidelines.

40) H.

This patient has chorioamnionitis at 34 weeks' gestation with an uncomplicated fetal tachycardia. However, with a closed cervical opening, an attempt at vaginal delivery is likely to be prolonged, further increasing the risk of fetal compromise. Intravenous antibiotics will not be the most appropriate immediate action.

2. Practice Paper 2: Questions

Option list for Questions 1–3

A.	Ascending from the genital tract
B.	Blood borne
C.	Breastfeeding
D.	Drinking contaminated milk
E.	Droplets
F.	Eating contaminated eggs
G.	Eating contaminated vegetables
H.	Eating soft cheese
I.	Faeco-oral transmission
J.	Female anopheles mosquito
K.	Hospital acquired
L.	Kissing infected persons
M.	Personal contact
N.	Prolonged personal contact
O.	Seeding of placenta with subsequent fetal transmission
P.	Sexual contact
Q.	Vertical transmission during delivery

Instructions: Select from the option list above the **single** most appropriate mode of transmission for each of the following infective organisms. Each mode of transmission may be selected once, more than once or not all.

G 1) *Taxoplasma gondii*

Q 2) Neonatal *Chlamydia trachomatis*.

H 3) *Listeria monocytogenes*.

Option list for Question 4

A.	Bacterial vaginosis
B.	*Chlamydia trachomatis*
C.	Chancroid
D.	Genital herpes
E.	Granuloma inguinale
F.	Human immunodeficiency virus
G.	Lymphogranuloma venereum
H.	Molluscum contagiosum
I.	*Mycoplasma genitalium*
J.	*Neisseria gonorrhoeae*
K.	Pediculosis
L.	Syphilis
M.	*Trichomonas vaginalis*
N.	Tropical ulcer
O.	Viral hepatitis
P.	*Ureaplasma urealyticum*

Instructions: The newborn baby described below presents within a week of vaginal delivery. Select from the option list above the **single** most likely sexually transmitted infection involved.

4) A newborn baby develops sticky eyes 5 days after a vaginal delivery. His mother did not have any vaginal discharge although she had experienced dysuria and frequency a few months before pregnancy. She was having regular sexual intercourse during pregnancy with her partner of 2 years' duration. On examination, both the baby's eyes are sticky and have a yellowish discharge. The conjunctiva is inflamed.

Option list for Questions 5–7

A.	Antibiotics and repair 3 months later
B.	Boari's flap
C.	Conservative management (leave alone)
D.	Cystoscopy and repair
E.	Diagnostic laparoscopy
F.	Diuretics
G.	Drain the air with a Verres needle
H.	Exploratory laparotomy
I.	Immediate fistula repair
J.	Indwelling catheter and antibiotics for 10 days
K.	Repair alone
L.	Repair and colostomy
M.	Repair and drain
N.	Repair and stent for 10 days
O.	Repair and indwelling catheter for 10 days
P.	Retrograde cystoureteroscopy
Q.	Stop the procedure, antibiotics and observe for 24 hours
R.	Ureteric implantation
S.	Ureteric stent
T.	Urethral catheter for 10 days

Instructions: The following patients developed complications that were recognized at the time of surgery. From the option list above, choose the **single** most appropriate immediate step that you will take to deal with the complication. Each option may be chosen once, more than once or not at all.

5) During Wertheim hysterectomy urine is observed to be coming through the patient's bladder. On further inspection, it is confirmed that there is a cut on the bladder.

6) A 30-year-old woman underwent laparoscopic surgical excision of extensive endometriosis 3 days ago. Following surgery she was found to have an increasing abdominal girth and pain. An intravenous urogram shows leakage of contrast from the left ureter.

A 7) A 46-year-old woman had an abdominal hysterectomy 4 days ago and is now complaining of continuous leaking of urine per vaginam. A dye test confirms that she has developed a vesicovaginal fistula and is understandably very distraught.

Option list for Question 8

A.	Amniocentesis for karyotype
B.	Amniocentesis for viral polymerase chain reaction (PCR)
C.	Biophysical profile
D.	Cardiotocograph (CTG)
E.	Computed tomography (CT) scan of the brain
F.	Detailed ultrasound scan
G.	Doppler of the middle cerebral artery
H.	Fetal blood sampling (FBS)
I.	Fetal electrocardiogram (ECG)
J.	Fetal haemoglobin electrophoresis
K.	Fetal blood group
L.	Magnetic resonance imaging (MRI) of brain
M.	Optical density of amniotic fluid
N.	Three-dimensional (3D) ultrasound scan
O.	Ultrasound scan for growth
P.	Uterine artery Doppler

Instructions: Select the **single** most appropriate fetal investigation from the option list above for the case scenarios described below.

G 8) A 24-year-old primigravida attends the fetal assessment unit for fetal assessment at 28 weeks' gestation on account of severe fetal growth restriction. The fundal height is 24 cm and amniotic fluid index is 5 cm (<5th centile for gestational age). The fetal heart rate auscultated with a Sonicaid is 168 bpm and described as having unprovoked decelerations.

Option list for Question 9

A.	Aqueous acetic acid application and biopsy
B.	Cervical cytology
C.	Colposcopy and biopsy of the vulva
D.	Colpophotography
E.	Endocervical swabs for sexually transmitted infections (STIs)
F.	Excisional biopsy
G.	Glucose tolerance test
H.	Liquid-based cytology
I.	Liver function test
J.	Punch biopsy
K.	Renal function test
L.	Serum vitamin B_{12} quantification
M.	Speculum examination
N.	Urinalysis
O.	Viral swabs from the low vagina

Instructions: The patient presented below was referred to a routine gynaecology clinic by her GP. Select from the option list above the **single** best first-line test to be undertaken to enable a diagnosis to be made.

J 9) A 50-year-old woman presents with red flat-topped lesions on the vulva and wrists. These were first noticed 4 months ago. They do not cause any discomfort but are embarrassing. On examination, she is found to have red/purple flat-topped nodular lesions and papules on the vulva. Similar lesions are identified on the wrist.

(L. planus)

Option list for Questions 10–12

A.	Appendicectomy
B.	Azithromycin
C.	Bowel resection
D.	Ceftraxone
E.	Cervical fibroid polypectomy
F.	Erythromicin
G.	Exploratory laparotomy
H.	Gentamicin
I.	Laparoscopic salpingectomy
J.	Opiate analgesics
K.	Oophorectomy
L.	Ovarian cystectomy
M.	Nasogastric tube and nil by mouth
N.	Nephrostomy
O.	Potent analgesics – non-opiates
P.	Reassurance
Q.	Rescan in 6 weeks
R.	Salpingectomy and fixing of the ovary
S.	Total abdominal hysterectomy and bilateral salpingo-oophorectomy
T.	Ultrasound-guided needle aspiration

Instructions: For each of the following case histories select the **single** most appropriate initial treatment option from the option list above. Each option may be chosen once, more than once or not at all.

10) A 20-year-old woman presents with a vaginal discharge, dysuria and right upper abdominal pain 1 week after unprotected sexual intercourse.

11) A 28-year-old woman presents with right-sided abdominal pain of 6 days' duration. The pain which was initially intermittent and later constant has now disappeared. An ultrasound examination suggests a dermoid cyst of the ovary. Her white cell count, which was high on admission, has now returned to normal.

12) A 50-year-old woman presents with an acute abdomen of 12 hours' duration. On examination she is found to have a tender abdomen with guarding and rebound. There is evidence of ascites. An ultrasound scan suggested a ruptured ovarian cyst.

Option list for Question 13

A.	Anaemia
B.	Anxiety
C.	Drug induced
D.	Domestic violence
E.	Ectopic beats
F.	Hyperglycaemia
G.	Hypoglycaemia
H.	Physiological
I.	Severe asthma
J.	Sinus tachycardia
K.	Stress
L.	Supraventricular tachycardia
M.	Thyrotoxicosis
N.	Phaeochromocytoma

Instructions: The patient described below presented with palpitations in pregnancy. Choose the **single** most likely cause of the palpitations from the option list above.

13) A 21-year-old immigrant who does not speak English is admitted with palpitations of 3 weeks' gestation. She has recently arrived in the country and is living with her husband's family. She is now 24 weeks pregnant. Nothing abnormal is found on examination.

Option list for Questions 14–15

A.	Adoption
B.	Bromocriptine
C.	Expectant management
D.	Follicle-stimulating hormone
E.	In vitro fertilization and embryo transfer (IVE-ET)
F.	Intrauterine insemination with husband's sperm
G.	Intrauterine insemination with donor sperm
H.	Intracytoplasmic sperm injection
I.	Orchidopexy
J.	Percutaneous sperm aspiration
K.	Reassurance
L.	Salpingotomy
M.	Sperm washing and insemination
N.	Steroids for antisperm antibodies
O.	Testosterone injections
P.	Varicolectomy
Q.	Vitamin E

Instructions: For each of the following cases of male infertility, select the **single** most appropriate initial treatment from the option list above. Each option may be selected once, more than once or not at all.

14) A couple attend the gynaecology outpatient department with primary infertility. Investigations reveal that the woman is ovulating normally and also has patent fallopian tubes. However, on examination the man is found to have small testicles and azoospermia.

15) A young couple attend with primary infertility of 3 years' duration. On investigation the woman is found to be ovulating and to have patent fallopian tubes at laparoscopy and dye testing. The man's semen analysis is normal.

Option list for Questions 16–18

A.	Bell's palsy (facial nerve palsy)
B.	Carpal tunnel syndrome
C.	Diabetes mellitus
D.	Epidural block
E.	Guillain–Barré syndrome
F.	Hyperventilation
G.	Lumbosacral trunk
H.	Meralgia paraesthetica (lateral cutaneous nerve of the thigh)
I.	Migraine
J.	Multiple sclerosis
K.	Transient ischaemic attacks
L.	Vitamin B_{12} deficiency

Instructions: For each of the following clinical scenarios, choose the **single** most likely cause of numbness from the option list above. Each option may be used once, more than once or not at all.

K 16) A 40-year-old G2P1 is seen at 24 weeks' gestation complaining of recurrent attacks of numbness in the left arm and forearm. She describes these as lasting for a few minutes to hours when they occur but usually no longer than 24 hours. There is no associated headache or dizziness. Occasionally these are preceded by blackouts that last a few seconds. Her blood sugars have been checked and found to be normal.

H 17) Mrs Jones is seen at 36 weeks' gestation in the antenatal clinic complaining of numbness and pain on the front and lateral aspect of her right thigh. This was of sudden onset and unassociated with any other precipitating factors or symptoms. On examination, her BP is 137/88 mmHg, pulse 86 bpm and fundal height 35 cm. There is a defined area of reduced sensation over L5 S1 and S2.

J 18) A 28-year-old G2P1 is seen at 27 weeks' gestation with numbness and pain on the front and side of the thigh (right) associated with paraesthesia. The symptoms have been intermittent up to now but she is worried that they may affect her pregnancy, although they have not become worse during the pregnancy. She has, on occasion, had double vision. On examination, her BP is 126/85 mmHg and the fundal height corresponds to gestation. There is increased spasticity in the muscles of the lower limb but nothing else abnormal.

Option list for Questions 19–20

A.	Basal body temperature
B.	Day 21 progesterone
C.	Endometrial biopsy
D.	Falloposcopy
E.	FSH and LH
F.	Hysteroscopy
G.	Hysterosalpingography
H.	Hysteroscopic contrast sonography (HyCoSy)
I.	In vitro mucus penetration test
J.	Laparoscopy and dye test
K.	Prolactin
L.	Postcoital test
M.	Salpingoscopy
N.	Spinnbarkeit
O.	Transvaginal ultrasound scan of the pelvis

Instructions: For each of the following case scenarios, select from the option list above the **single** most informative initial investigation that you will perform on the patient. Each investigation may be selected once, more than once or not at all.

K 19) A 26-year-old woman presents with infertility, headaches and an occasional discharge from the breast. She had a fracture to her skull 2 years ago.

G 20) A 26-year-old woman presents with primary infertility of 2 years' duration. She was investigated in her native country 2 years ago and had a dilatation and curettage. Since then her periods have become light, although they are still regular. Her husband's semen is normal.

Option list for Questions 21–22

A.	Alcoholic liver cirrhosis
B.	Bronchial carcinoma
C.	Bronchiectasis
D.	Chronic suppurative lung disease
E.	Congenital cyanotic heart disease
F.	Cryptogenic fibrosing alveolitis
G.	Empyema
H.	Infective endocarditis
I.	Inflammatory bowel disease
J.	Liver abscess
K.	Lung abscess
L.	Mesothelioma
M.	Pleural effusion
N.	Squamous cell carcinoma
O.	Tuberculosis

Instructions: For each of the patients below, chose the **single** most appropriate diagnosis from the option list above. Each option may be selected once, more than once or not at all.

21) A 38-year-old woman, who worked in an ammunitions factory during the Iraq war, presents to her GP at 27 weeks' gestation with abdominal pain, constipation, polyuria, haemoptysis and weight loss. A chest X-ray taken 3 years ago showed multiple pleural plaques only.

22) A 32-year-old woman present to her GP at 26 weeks' gestation with dyspnoea. On examination, she is cyanosed and mildly dyspnoeic at rest, with fine late inspiratory crackles heard bilaterally in the chest.

Option list for Questions 23–25

A.	Anticardiolipin antibodies
B.	Anti-thrombin III
C.	Autoimmune profile
D.	Diagnostic laparoscopy
E.	Fasting homocysteine
F.	Follicle-stimulating hormone
G.	Full blood count
H.	Hystero-contrast sonography
I.	Hysterosalpingography
J.	Hysteroscopy
K.	Luteinizing hormone
L.	Oral glucose tolerance test
M.	Protein S
N.	Thyroid function test
O.	Thyroid peroxidase antibodies
P.	Ultrasound of the pelvis

Instructions: You are seeing the following patients with a history of recurrent miscarriages in the gynaecology clinic. Select from the option list above the **single** most informative immediate investigation that you will request. Each option may be selected once, more than once or not at all.

23) A 27-year-old woman with three miscarriages is seen in the gynaecology clinic 6 weeks after her third pregnancy. Her periods have always been irregular but she is not overweight. She does not tolerate the cold weather very well but states that she has always been like this as far as she can remember.

24) A 30 year old is seen in the clinic 3 months after her fourth miscarriage. The first was at 8 weeks' gestation after which she had an evacuation. The next three occurred at 5.5, 7 and 6 weeks, respectively. Her periods are regular and her BMI is 20 kg/m^2.

25) A 22-year-old female teacher who has had three miscarriages all in the first trimester is seen in the clinic. She is obese, has become increasingly lethargic and is intolerant of cold. Her periods are irregular and she suffers from hirsutism.

Option list for Questions 26–27

A.	Antibiotics and deliver
B.	ARM
C.	Breech extraction
D.	Cardiotocograph
E.	Ductus venosus Doppler
F.	Elective caesarean section
G.	Emergency caesarean section
H.	Fetal blood sampling
I.	Forceps delivery
J.	General anaesthesia caesarean section
K.	Induction of labour
L.	Intrauterine transfusion
M.	Left lateral position and oxygen by facemask
N.	Middle cerebral artery Doppler
O.	Steroids
P.	Syntocinon infusion
Q.	Terbutaline – subcutaneous
R.	Ventouse delivery

Instructions: For each of the cases described below choose the **single** most appropriate first-line treatment from the option list above. Each option may be used once, more than once or not at all.

26) A 38-year-old woman with twins at 37 weeks' gestation was admitted in spontaneous labour at 9 cm dilatation. She quickly progressed to full dilatation and delivered the first twin without any complications. Soon after there was a brisk vaginal loss followed by a bradycardia of the second twin.

27) A 20-year-old primigravida is seen in the clinic at 26 weeks' gestation with a suspected growth-restricted fetus. The fundal height measured 23 cm. An ultrasound scan was performed and the fetal measurements were approximately equal to that of a 22-week fetus. The amniotic fluid index was above the 10th centile and the umbilical artery Doppler was normal.

Option list for Questions 28–30

A.	Anterior exenteration
B.	Bilateral salpingo-oophorectomy
C.	Chemotherapy
D.	Cone biopsy
E.	Excision biopsy
F.	5-Fluorouracil
G.	Palliative care
H.	Posterior exenteration
I.	Progestogen therapy
J.	Radical vulvectomy
K.	Radiotherapy
L.	Regular follow-ups
M.	Simple vulvectomy
N.	Total abdominal hysterectomy
O.	Total abdominal hysterectomy and bilateral salpingo-oophorectomy
P.	Total vaginectomy
Q.	Wertheim's hysterectomy

Instructions: The following patients presented to the gynaecology oncology clinic. Choose the **single** most effective treatment from the option list above. Each option may be selected once, more than once or not at all.

28) A 78-year-old woman presents with a single ulcer on the vulva. It was first noticed 4 months ago but it recently started bleeding. A biopsy of the ulcer is sent for histology which is reported as carcinoma. There is no node involvement.

29) A 23-year-old woman is found to have to have persistently rising human chorionic gonadotrophin levels 6 months after an evacuation of a complete molar pregnancy. She complained of abdominal pain and an ultrasound revealed bilateral ovarian cysts each measuring 7.6 cm.

30) A 30-year-old woman with a severely dyskaryotic cervical smear, which was reported to contain malignant cells, is found to have carcinoma of the cervix stage IB. Although her family is incomplete she considers her health to be paramount.

Option list for Questions 31–32

A.	Amniocentesis for culture
B.	Amniocentesis for PCR
C.	Blood culture
D.	Blood film
E.	Chorionic villous sampling
F.	Culture of amniotic fluid
G.	Fetal blood sampling
H.	Fetal liver biopsy
I.	Immediate viral immunoglobulin G (IgG) quantification
J.	IgG antibodies in maternal blood to determine susceptibility
K.	IgG antibodies
L.	Immunoglobulin M quantification in maternal blood
M.	Magnetic resonance imaging
N.	Ultrasound scan
O.	Urine microscopy, culture and sensitivity
P.	Sputum culture
Q.	Viral PCR in maternal urine

Instructions: From the option list above, select the **single** most suitable first-line diagnostic test to help counsel the patient or confirm that either she or her fetus has the suspected infection. Each option may be selected once, more than once or not at all.

31) Mrs C is a school teacher in week 15 of her pregnancy. She had her booking blood test 2 weeks ago. She recently had contacts with a child who was described as having German measles. Although she has not developed any symptoms yet, she is worried about the risks of this infection to her baby.

32) A 40-year-old woman who underwent infertility treatment is now 27 weeks pregnant. She is very worried that she may have toxoplasmosis as she has recently returned from southern France where she ate a lot of poorly cooked meat. She complains of vague generalized symptoms.

Option list for Questions 33–35

A.	Alfa-fetoprotein (AFP)
B.	β-Human chorionic gonadotrophin (βhCG)
C.	*BRCA-1* and *BRCA-2*
D.	CA-125
E.	Cervical smear
F.	Colposcopy
G.	Cytology of peritoneal lavage
H.	Cytobrush
I.	Doppler of the ovarian vessels
J.	Endometrial biopsy
K.	Examination under anaesthesia
L.	Hysteroscopy
M.	Human papillomavirus (HPV) screening
N.	Intravenous antibiotics
O.	Omental biopsy
P.	Risk malignancy index
Q.	Thyroid function test
R.	Ultrasound scan of the pelvis

Instructions: For each of the following case scenarios, choose the **single** most useful investigation that you will undertake from the option list above. Each option may be selected once, more than once or not at all.

33) A 54-year-old G2P1 presents with postmenopausal bleeding of 3 months' duration. Her periods had always been irregular and her two previous pregnancies were conceived on clomifene citrate.

34) A 36-year-old HIV-positive woman, who had never been to the doctor before, presented with anxieties about genital malignancies. She had four children, all by different partners, and is currently not in a stable relationship. Her last period was 3 months ago.

35) A 45-year-old teacher presented for investigations in view of her family history. Her mother and aunt died of ovarian cancer. She had been on the pill since the age of 16 years and only came off to have her two children.

Option list for Questions 36–38

A.	Antibiotics – intravenous
B.	Anticoagulation – full
C.	Elective caesarean section
D.	Emergency caesarean section
E.	Induction of labour
F.	Intramuscular opiates
G.	Intravenous fluids
H.	Intravenous fluids and thromboprophylaxis
I.	Intravenous fluids, antibiotics and thromboprophylaxis
J.	Lumbar epidural
K.	Middle cerebral artery Doppler
L.	Steroids
M.	Thrombolysis
N.	Thromboprophylaxis
O.	Transfusion with red cells
P.	Umbilical artery Doppler
Q.	Transfusion with whole blood

Instructions: For each of the following clinical scenarios, choose the **single** most appropriate intervention from the option list above. Each intervention may be selected once, more than once or not at all.

36) A 23-year-old woman, known to have sickle cell anaemia (HbSS), presents in her first pregnancy at 34 weeks' gestation feeling generally unwell. The fundal height measures 32 cm.

On examination she is found to have a mild temperature and a blood pressure of 140/65 mmHg. There is nitrites + and protein + in her urine. Her haemoglobin is 8.7 g/dL.

37) A 27-year-old woman, known to have sickle cell anaemia (HbSC), presents at 34 weeks with nausea and vomiting of 3 days' duration. On examination, her temperature is 36.9°C, her pulse is 82 bpm and her blood pressure is 110/65 mmHg. The uterine fundus measures 32 cm, the lie of the fetus is longitudinal and CTG is normal. The cervix is closed. Urinalysis reveals nitrites +, leucocytes +, proteins +. Her haemoglobin is 7.5 g/dL.

38) A 29-year-old G3P0 presents at 37 weeks with absent fetal movements of 24 hours' duration. On examination, the fundal height is 36 cm and the lie is longitudinal with cephalic presentation. The uterus is soft and the CTG shows reduced baseline variability with neither accelerations nor decelerations after 30 minutes. A biophysical profile was undertaken and the score is 6.

Option list for Questions 39–40

A.	Abdominal aorta
B.	Deep circumflex iliac artery
C.	External iliac artery
D.	External pudendal artery
E.	Inferior epigastric artery
F.	Inferior rectal artery
G.	Inferior vesical artery
H.	Iliolumbar artery
I.	Internal iliac artery
J.	Internal pudendal artery
K.	Lateral sacral artery
L.	Left ovarian vein
M.	Left renal artery
N.	Middle rectal artery
O.	Obliterated umbilical artery
P.	Obturator artery
Q.	Pampiniform plexus of veins
R.	Right ovarian artery
S.	Right renal artery
T.	Superficial circumflex iliac artery
U.	Superior epigastric artery
V.	Superior mesenteric artery
W.	Superior vesical artery
X.	Uterine artery

Instructions: Below are descriptions of vessels that the gynaecologist often encounters during surgery. For each of the descriptions, select from the option list above the **single** most appropriate vessel that fits this description. Each option may be selected once, more than once or not at all.

B 39) During a Burch colposuspension, the surgeon notices torrential bleeding in the retropubic space. The bleeding is thought to be arterial and resulted from an injury to a blood vessel during dissection close to the bony pelvic wall.

40) A three-portal laparoscopic diathermy to endometriosis was performed on a 26-year-old woman with primary infertility. The procedure was described as uncomplicated, but she collapsed 3 hours later and was rushed back to theatre. She was found to have one litre of blood in her abdomen but there was no obvious bleeding vessel in the peritoneal cavity.

2. Practice Paper 2: Answers

1) G.
Eating contaminated vegetables or poorly cooked beef is the main route by which *Toxoplasma gondii* is transmitted.

2) Q.
Neonatal *Chlamydia trachomatis* is acquired through the genital tract during delivery. It tends to present approximately 5 days after delivery.

3) H.
Listeria monocytogenes is commonly transmitted through eating soft cheese and eggs.

4) B.
The baby presented with symptoms 5 days after a vaginal delivery. The most likely cause of the conjunctivitis is *Chlamydia trachomatis*. Other causes of neonatal conjunctivitis such as *Neisseria gonorrhoeae* tend to present approximately 3 days after delivery.

5) O.
Any bladder injury recognized at the time of surgery should be repaired and the bladder rested for at least 7 days. Whether prophylactic antibiotics should be offered at the same time is debatable. However, the general consensus is that, with an indwelling catheter and a repair, the patients is more likely to benefit from antibiotics. None of the options given combines this ideal treatment. The closest one is repair and indwelling catheter for 10 days.

6) S.
The ureter in this patient should be stented. The duration of the stenting should be determined by the urologist. The fact that she is presenting with an increasing abdominal girth will suggest that this was not immediately recognized. Primary repair of the injury before stenting is therefore an option that will not be ideal. Whether or not a repair is offered at a later stage will depend on several factors, one of which will be the spontaneous healing of the ureter when the stent is removed.

7) A.
Repair of a vesicovaginal fistula is not recommended until the tissues around the fistula have become less oedematous and infected. Therefore, the option is antibiotics and repair 3 months later.

8) G.

This fetus is severely growth restricted and a decision needs to be made on the timing of delivery. Doppler testing of the middle cerebral artery will identify the centralization of blood flow in a severely compromised fetus. A biophysical profile is useful but will not be as informative as a Doppler of the middle cerebral artery. Fetal blood sampling, however, will allow for karyotyping and the determination of blood gases, is invasive and carries significant risks, which at 28 weeks' gestation are greater than the risks of delivery.

9) J.

A punch biopsy will allow for a histological diagnosis of the pathology. A colposcopy and biopsy will provide the same information, but the value of a colposcopy in this patient is questionable. The most likely diagnosis is lichen planus.

10) B.

The most likely diagnosis for this patient is infection with *Chlamydia trachomatis*. Although there are several treatment options, a single course of azithromycin is an effective treatment that lasts for days. The advantage of this option is the elimination of the effect of compliance on efficacy.

11) K.

The history presented is typical of ovarian torsion. By the time the pain has disappeared, the ovary is no longer viable. Whether this procedure is performed laparoscopically or by laparotomy will depend on the expertise available.

12) O.

The cyst has already ruptured. Therefore, the best option is symptomatic treatment with potent analgesics and observation. There is no need for intervention unless the symptoms fail to respond.

13) K.

The features with which the patient presents are symptomatic of stress. Although thyrotoxicosis, anaemia and ectopic beats can all present with similar features, there are factors in her history that make stress more likely.

14) G.

The small testicles and azoospermia would suggest that spermatogenesis is not taking place within the testes. Spermatid aspiration for ICSI is therefore not an option. The only way that this couple can achieve a pregnancy is by using donated sperms. These can be used as part of either an IVF programme or a donor insemination programme. The latter is less expensive and has a success rate that is comparable to that of IVF-ET.

15) C.

This couple have unexplained infertility. Expectant management has been shown to be associated with a high pregnancy rate over a period of time. As this couple are young, this would be the best option to offer together with counselling.

16) K.

The symptoms are transient, making the diagnosis simple. However, hyperventilation must be considered a differential diagnosis.

17) H.

Meralgia paraesthetica is an uncommon presentation in obstetrics but the location of the signs when this patient was examined provides the clues to this being the most likely cause of her symptoms.

18) J.

Multiple sclerosis (MS) is rare at this age, but the symptoms and signs point to this diagnosis. The increased spasticity in the lower limbs with associated abnormality would either indicate MS or a spinal lesion. There are no features of a spinal lesion in this patient which thus leaves MS as the most likely diagnosis.

19) K.

Infertility and headaches will suggest an intracranial lesion as the possible cause of the infertility. The occasional discharge from the breast points to hyperprolactinaemia and this can be excluded by measuring the serum prolactin.

20) G.

The most likely diagnosis in this patient is Asherman's syndrome. This can be diagnosed either by hysteroscopy or hysterosalpingography (HSG). The advantage of performing an HSG is that the tubes will also be examined whereas a hysteroscopy will not investigate tubal patency.

21) L.

From the information provided, mesothelioma is the likely diagnosis. Although it may be possible that she has cryptogenic fibrosing alveolitis or squamous cell carcinoma, this is not a typical picture of these conditions.

22) E.

Central cyanosis associated with crepitations in both lung fields indicates a cardiac condition — either acquired or congenital. The only diagnostic options for this patient are, therefore, either infective endocarditis or cyanotic heart disease. Since endocarditis does not typically present with bilateral crackles in the chest, the only option is therefore congenital cyanotic heart disease.

23) P.

The most likely causes of the symptoms are hypothyroidism and polycystic ovary syndrome. However, the recurrent miscarriages and irregular periods associated with the symptoms of thyroid dysfunction from which the patient has indicated she had always suffered would suggest that PCOS should be excluded first. An ultrasound of the pelvis will be the most informative method for the diagnosis of PCOS. None of the other biochemical investigations will provide more information than an ultrasound scan.

24) J.

The patient's history suggests that a cause of the miscarriages is related to the evacuation performed after the first miscarriage. A hysteroscopy will be the most informative diagnostic test as it will identify intrauterine adhesions and fibrosis, which are pathognomonic of Asherman's syndrome.

25) N.

Obesity, irregular periods and hirsutism are all features of PCOS. Increasing lethargy will suggest hypothyroidism or Cushing's syndrome. However, intolerance of cold and increasing lethargy are highly suggestive of a thyroid dysfunction. Hypothyroidism is therefore the diagnosis that should first be excluded and for this a thyroid function is required.

26) J.

This is an emergency and requires immediate delivery. A caesarean section under general anaesthetic is the best option as there is no time either to top up the epidural or to give her a spinal epidural. As no information is provided about the lie and position of the fetus, an instrumental delivery, though a possibility, is not the most appropriate option for this patient.

27) H.

A fetal blood sample will enable karyotyping, estimation of blood gases and fetal haemoglobin, as well as providing an opportunity to screen for infections that may be responsible for the early onset fetal growth restriction. A normal amniotic fluid volume and severe fetal growth restriction suggest a high risk of karyotypic abnormality. Although delivery is an option, the approach to delivering the baby and the impact of the uterine scar on future fertility would require a less interventionist approach unless the fetus is known to be karyotypically normal.

28) M.

A simple vulvectomy will normally be considered adequate surgery for vulval carcinoma where there is no node involvement. Extensive surgery is recommended where there is sentinel node involvement.

29) C.

The βhCG levels should have returned to normal within this time period or have fallen significantly. Persistently high levels are an indication for the commencement of chemotherapy. Although this patient has bilateral ovarian cysts, they are likely to be theca lutein cysts and should be treated with chemotherapy rather than excision.

30) Q.

Surgery or radiotherapy for this stage of carcinoma of the cervix is associated with the same prognosis. However, at this young age, surgery offers significant advantages over radiotherapy. A cone biopsy would be inadequate at this stage.

31) J.

Immunization conveys life-long immunity, although approximately 3% of women will remain seronegative despite vaccination. The presence of IgG antibodies in the serum will suggest previous infections. If she gives a history of immunization then she can be reassured that the first option will be to determine the presence of IgG antibodies in her blood (if stored).

32) J.

Susceptibility will depend on the presence or absence of antibodies to *Toxoplasma gondii* in the maternal blood. If she has been exposed to protozoa in the past, she will have protection. However, if not, then she will be at risk. A blood sample for the determination of IgG antibodies will determine her susceptibility.

33) J.

The most important pathology that needs to be excluded is endometrial cancer or atypical hyperplasia. Based on the patient's history, the risk of her having any of these pathologies is considerably high. The gold standard for this investigation is biopsy. An ultrasound scan for endometrial thickness will not exclude pathology but will identify those at risk who will therefore require an endometrial biopsy.

34) E.

HIV-positive women are at an increased risk of cervical carcinoma and increased risk of HPV infection because of their reduced immunity. A cervical smear is therefore the investigation of choice. A colposcopy is not indicated for this woman.

35) C.

The only current reliable screening test to identify women at risk of ovarian cancer is genetic screening for *BRCA* genes. A family history is essential for genetic screening. Two relatives of this patient died from ovarian cancer and therefore she meets the criteria for testing. Whether tissues are available for screening is uncertain.

36) I.
The most likely problems in this patient are urinary tract infections and pseudotoxaemia of pregnancy. Pseudotoxaemia is characterized by systolic hypertension and proteinuria, and typically occurs in women with sickle cell anaemia. Bone marrow embolism is the most dreaded complication. Therefore, in this patient a combination of intravenous fluids, antibiotics and thromboprophylaxis would be the most suitable treatment option. Once the diagnosis is suspected, the baby should be delivered.

37) I.
The most likely cause of these symptoms is urinary tract infections. The vomiting and pyrexia will increase the risk of venous thromboembolism. Intravenous antibiotics and thromboprophylaxis are therefore the best treatment options.

38) E.
A biophysical profile score of less than 8 indicates delivery. This patient is at 37 weeks' gestation and fetal growth is normal. A CTG with reduced baseline variability after 30 minutes, associated with a history of absent fetal movements, is suggestive of delivery; for this patient, there is no contraindication for an induced vaginal delivery.

39) B.
Deep circumflex iliac artery.

40) E.
Inferior epigastric artery is the only likely source of the bleeding and the injury would have occurred during the introduction of the third port. Tamponade by the instrument through this port would have stemmed the bleeding until the port was removed and the incision closed.

3. Practice Paper 3: Questions

Option list for Questions 1–2

A.	Amniocentesis for culture
B.	Amniocentesis for PCR
C.	Blood culture
D.	Blood film
E.	Chorionic villous sampling
F.	Culture of amniotic fluid
G.	Fetal blood sampling
H.	Fetal liver biopsy
I.	IgG in stored blood
J.	Immediate IgG quantification in a fresh blood sample
K.	IgM quantification in maternal blood and repeat in 10–14 days if negative
L.	MRI
M.	Ultrasound scan
N.	Urine microscopy, culture and sensitivity
O.	Sputum culture
P.	Viral PCR in urine

Instructions: From the option list above, select the **single** most suitable diagnostic test to confirm that either the patient or her fetus has the suspected infection. Each option may be selected once, more than once or not at all.

1) Mrs C, a school teacher who recently arrived from South Africa in week 15 of her pregnancy, has had contact with a child in her school described as having red cheeks and a running nose. Although she has not yet developed any symptoms, she is worried about the risks of infection to her baby.

P 2) A 24-year-woman, who underwent infertility treatment, delivered a symmetrically small baby at 40 weeks' gestation. The baby has hepatosplenomegaly and petechiae all over its body. It is suspected that the mother may have had cytomegalovirus infection in pregnancy.

Option list for Questions 3–4

A.	Aciclovir
B.	Azithromycin
C.	Benzylpenicillin
D.	Cephalexin
E.	Clotrimazole
F.	Cryotherapy
G.	Erythromycin
H.	Gamma-benzene hexachloride
I.	Highly active antiretroviral treatment (HAART)
J.	Metronidazole
K.	Ofloxacin
L.	Podophyllotoxin
M.	Procaine penicillin
N.	Spectinomycin
O.	Vaginal clindamycin

Instructions: The patients described below have a sexually transmitted infection. Select from the option list above the **single** most suitable first-line treatment. Each option may be selected once, more than once or not at all.

B 3) A 16-year-old girl presents with right iliac fossa abdominal pain, irregular periods and a vaginal discharge. Her last period was 5 weeks ago. She is not on any form of contraception and her periods have always been irregular (occurring every 4–7 weeks). On examination she was found to be very tender in the lower abdomen. Cervical motion tenderness was positive. A diagnostic laparoscopy showed widespread inflammatory changes in the pelvis, especially on the fallopian tubes and pelvic peritoneum. The perihepatic area was also severely inflamed.

4) A 21-year-old woman presents with lumps on the vulva which were first noticed 2 weeks ago. They are non-itchy but uncomfortable. There is no associated vaginal discharge. Her last menstrual period was 1 week ago. On examination she is found to have widespread discrete whitish lesions on the vulva and perineum extending to the perianal area.

Option list for Questions 5–6

A.	Anti-rho antibody
B.	Bronchoscopy for PCR
C.	CA-125
D.	Cardiac echo
E.	Chest X-ray
F.	C-reactive protein
G.	Computed tomography scan of the brain
H.	Electrocardiogram (ECG)
I.	Electroencephalogram (EEG)
J.	Fibrinogen degradation products
K.	Four-point blood glucose
L.	Free thyroxine (FT$_4$)
M.	Glycated haemoglobin
N.	Mantoux test
O.	Oral glucose tolerance test
P.	Random blood glucose
Q.	Renal ultrasound
R.	Respiratory peak flow volume
S.	Thyroid-stimulating hormone
T.	24-hour ECG tape
U.	24-hour urinary protein
V.	Urea ultrasound scan – M-mode and electrolytes

Instructions: One of the patients described below presents in the second trimester of pregnancy and the other presents in the first trimester. Choose from the option list above the **single** most useful test to assess the severity of the conditions with which they present.

R 5) A 20-year-old asthmatic woman presents at 16 weeks' gestation to the maternal medicine clinic. She is currently taking beta-sympathomimetics, which are thought to be controlling her asthma suboptimally. On examination, she is comfortable at rest although has mild rhonchi bilaterally.

B 6) A 30-year-old mother of three complains of chronic cough and chest pains associated with breathlessness and night sweats at 10 weeks' gestation. She also complaints of palpitations, listlessness and occasional headaches. Her 3-year-old child was recently diagnosed with pulmonary tuberculosis.

Option list for Questions 7–9

A.	Bowel preparation
B.	Chest X-ray
C.	ECG
D.	Endocervical swab for *Chlamydia trachomatis*
E.	Examine under anaesthesia and cystoscopy
F.	Full blood count
G.	Group and save
H.	Haemoglobin electrophoresis
I.	Obtain consent
J.	Pregnancy test
K.	Proctosigmoidoscopy
L.	Thrombophilia screen
M.	Ultrasound scan of the abdomen
N.	Urea and electrolytes
O.	Ultrasound scan of the pelvis
P.	Urinalysis and midstream urine for microscopy and sensitivity if indicated

Instructions: The following patients are being prepared for surgery. Select the **single** most relevant unique investigation that you will perform prior to surgery from the option list above. Each option may be selected once, more than once or not at all.

E 7) A 29-year-old woman who has just been diagnosed with carcinoma of the cervix, confirmed after a colposcopic directed biopsy, is being scheduled for Wertheim's hysterectomy.

M 8) A 37-year-old woman presented with an abdominal mass arising from the pelvis and extending up to the umbilicus. On examination the mass is clinically thought to be multiple uterine fibroids. The patient is placed on the waiting list for an abdominal hysterectomy.

P 9) A 56-year-old diabetic woman is scheduled to have a vaginal hysterectomy and an anterior repair because of a second-degree uterine descent and a moderate cystocele.

Option list for Questions 10–12

A.	Amnioinfusion
B.	Amnioreduction
C.	Antibiotics – erythromycin
D.	Deliver – induction of labour
E.	Drainage of ascites and/or pleural effusion
F.	Dexamethasone/betamethasone
G.	Digoxin
H.	Elective caesarean section
I.	Gene therapy
J.	Hyperbaric oxygen
K.	Intrauterine transfusion
L.	Laser division of chorionic plate vessels
M.	Non-steroidal anti-inflammatory agents (NSAIDs), e.g. indometacin
N.	Selective feticide
O.	Selective feticide and delivery
P.	Septotomy
Q.	Termination of pregnancy
R.	Urethral catheterization
S.	Vesicoperitoneal shunt
T.	Antibiotics and deliver

Instructions: For each of the clinical scenarios presented below, choose the **single** most suitable treatment option from the option list above. Each option may be selected once, more than once or not at all.

T **10)** A 30-year-old primigravida attends at 33 weeks' gestation with a history suspicious of rupture of fetal membranes 24 hours previously. She has had a constant discharge which was initially clear but is now yellowish. On examination, her temperature is 37.6°C, pulse 92 bpm and BP 116/82 mmHg. The fundal height is 31 cm and the uterus is irritable but soft. Fetal CTG is reactive and normal. A copious discharge is confirmed on speculum examination. Her white cell count is 16 000 and her C-reactive protein is 48.

C **11)** A 40-year-old G2P0 attends triage at 32 weeks with a suspected rupture of fetal membranes. This is her second admission: the first was at 26 weeks with antepartum haemorrhage and at that visit she was given dexamethasone. An ultrasound scan shows a normal fetus with oligohydramnios.

O **12)** A 24-year-old woman presents at 30 weeks' gestation with reduced fetal movements. She has twins conceived naturally but missed her detailed ultrasound scan when she travelled to Asia. An ultrasound scan shows one fetus to be normal and the other to have a hypoplasic right ventricle.

Option list for Questions 13–14

A.	Acute contact dermatitis
B.	Benign mucous membrane pemphigoid
C.	Contact dermatitis
D.	Diabetic vulvitis
E.	Dysaesthetic vulvodynia
F.	Hydradenitis suppurativa
G.	Lichen planus
H.	Lichen sclerosus
I.	Lichen simplex (eczema)
J.	Malignant melanoma
K.	Paget's disease
L.	Psoriasis
M.	Vulval carcinoma
N.	Vulval Crohn's disease
O.	Vulval intraepithelial neoplasia
P.	Vulval vestibulitis syndrome
Q.	Zoon's vulvitis

Instructions: For each of the following clinical conditions, select the **single most likely diagnosis** from the option list above. Each option may be selected once, more than once or not at all.

13) A 32-year-old woman presents with extensive ulcers on the vulva and a dirty brown vaginal discharge of 7 months' duration. The discharge is intermittent. The ulcerations are widespread and are associated with significant scarring.

14) A 43 year old presents with troublesome itching of the vulva of 12 months' duration. She was sterilized 7 years ago and her last cervical smear was 2 years ago. On examination, her vulva is found to have multiple, red, crusted plaques with sharp edges. No other pelvic abnormality is identified.

Option list for Questions 15–18

A.	Angina
B.	Anxiety induced
C.	Aortic dissecting aneurysm
D.	Gastro-oesophageal reflux
E.	Ischaemic heart disease
F.	Musculoskeletal
G.	Myocardiac infarction
H.	Pleural effusion
I.	Pneumonia
J.	Pneumothorax
K.	Pulmonary embolism
L.	Subcostal neuralgia

Instructions: For each of the following clinical scenarios, select the **single** most likely cause of the chest pain from the option list above. Each option may be used once, more than once or not at all.

15) A 39-year-old woman, who smokes 20 cigarettes a day, presents at 35 weeks' gestation with sudden-onset chest pain which is central and radiating to the neck. The pain, which she has had for the past 2 days, is made worse by exercise. Her BP is 140/90 mmHg, pulse 106 bpm and the fundal height is 34 cm. Serum troponin is elevated.

16) A 40-year-old woman is seen in triage with severe pain radiating to the back at 36 weeks' gestation. The pain is associated with systolic hypertension. She gives a family history of Marfan's syndrome in her sister. On examination, her BP is 160/80 mmHg and her pulse is 114 bpm. There is a murmur consistent with aortic regurgitation.

17) A 29-year-old primigravida presents at 28 weeks' gestation with a right-sided chest pain which is worse on deep inspiration. There is an associated cough, mild pyrexia and breathlessness. On examination, her temperature is 37.6°C, BP is 150/90 mmHg and pulse is 102 bpm. The trachea is central and the chest is symmetrical. Her white cell count is 23×10^9/L.

18) At 41 weeks a 40-year-old woman had a spontaneous vaginal delivery of a healthy female weighing 4.3 kg. Soon after delivery, she developed a left-sided pleuritic chest pain associated with breathlessness.

Option list for Questions 19–21

A.	Bilateral absence of the vas deferens
B.	Cryptorchidism
C.	Diabetes mellitus
D.	Genital tract obstruction
E.	Genital tuberculosis
F.	Idiopathic semen quality impairment
G.	Immunological disorders – sperms coated with antibodies
H.	Immotile cilia syndrome
I.	Kallmann's syndrome
J.	Klinefelter's syndrome
K.	Male accessory gland infection
L.	Orchitis
M.	Occupational factors
N.	Retrograde ejaculation
O.	Sulfasalazine
P.	Varicocele

Instructions: The following men have attended an infertility clinic with their partners. Investigations have confirmed that the men are the cause of the infertility. Select the **single** most likely cause of their infertility from the option list above. Each option may be selected once, more than once or not al all.

19) A 27-year-old, 2.1 m tall man attends with his wife for infertility. The wife has a normal ovulatory cycle and patent fallopian tubes at laparoscopy. The man confirms that he is very aggressive and has very little interest in sex. His testicles are on the small size.

20) A man had a semen analysis as part of investigations for infertility which showed asthenozoospermia. A subsequent mixed antiglobulin reaction (MAR) test was positive.

H 21) A 40-year-old man is investigated with his wife for secondary infertility. His semen analysis showed asthenozoospermia. He has been suffering from chronic productive cough and sinusitis for the past 2 years.

Option list for Questions 22–24

A.	Admit for monitoring
B.	Amniodrainage
C.	Amnioinfusion
D.	Atosiban
E.	Cervical cerclage
F.	Corticosteroids
G.	CTG monitoring
H.	Delivery
I.	Emergency caesarean section
J.	Foley's catheter and cervical cerclage
K.	In utero transfer
L.	Intravenous antibiotics
M.	Laser division of chorionic plate vessels
N.	Middle cerebral artery (MCA) Doppler
O.	Oral erythromycin
P.	Regular ultrasound scans
Q.	Regular transvaginal cervical length measurement
R.	Selective feticide
S.	Septotomy
T.	Termination of pregnancy
U.	Umbilical artery Doppler

Instructions: For each of the clinical cases described below, choose the **single** most likely management option from the option list above. Each option may be selected once, more than once or not at all.

22) A 28-year-old woman attends triage with tightening at 26 weeks' gestation. The hospital is a level II unit for neonatal care. On examination she is found to have a 3 cm dilated cervix and bulging membranes. The CTG is normal and there are no obvious contractions on the trace.

? see answer

H 23) A 30-year-old woman with a dichorionic diamniotic twin pregnancy is seen in a small district hospital at 36 weeks' gestation. An ultrasound scan for growth shows that both twins are growth restricted: the first measures approximately 32 weeks' gestation and the second approximately 34 weeks' gestation. The liquor volume is reduced in both twins.

T 24) A 30-year-old women attended for her booking for antenatal care at 11 weeks' gestation. An ultrasound scan showed a monochorionic monoamniotic twin pregnancy. At 20 weeks' gestation, when she attended for her detailed scan, one of the twins was dead. The fetal anatomy of the surviving twin was normal except for areas of cerebromalacia in both cerebral ventricles.

Option list for Questions 25–29

A.	Adenomyosis
B.	Chronic renal failure
C.	Cushing's syndrome
D.	Dysfunctional uterine bleeding
E.	Endometrial hyperplasia
F.	Endometrial polyps
G.	Endometriosis
H.	Factor X deficiency
I.	Hyperthyroidism
J.	Hypothyroidism
K.	Idiopathic thrombocytopenic purpura (ITP)
L.	Intrauterine contraceptive device
M.	Pelvic inflammatory disease
N.	Polycystic ovary syndrome
O.	Uterine fibroids
P.	Von Willebrand's disease

Instructions: For each of the clinical scenarios presented below, choose the **single** most likely cause of menstrual dysfunction from the option list above. Each option may be selected once, more than once or not at all.

M 25) A 24-year-old woman presents with heavy and painful periods of 3 years' duration. She experiences significant throbbing in the pelvis premenstrually and during menstruation. Her pains tend to remain as a dull sensation after the first few days. On examination, her BMI is 28 kg/m^2, the uterus is anteverted, fixed and tender, and cervical motion tenderness is positive on both adnexa. Her hormone profile is as follows: prolactin = 497 mIU/L, FSH = 6.3 IU/L, LH = 5.7 IU/L, TSH = 3.1 IU/L, free T$_4$ = 15 pmol/L.

G 26) A 35-year-old woman presents with heavy periods of 4 years' duration. Her abdomen has also been swelling for the past 7 months to the extent that her clothes are not fitting properly. She is nulliparous and has tried unsuccessfully to become pregnant. On examination her BMI is 27 kg/m^2 and there is a mass arising from the pelvis to midway between the symphysis pubis and the umbilicus. A pelvic examination confirmed the presence of a pelvic mass and indurated uterosacrals. An ultrasound scan shows bilateral enlarged ovaries contained areas of mixed echogenicity. The uterus is also enlarged and contains a few subserous fibroids. Her hormone profile is as follows: prolactin = 608 mIU/L, FSH = 6.3 IU/L, LH = 4.5 IU/L, TSH = 1.4 IU/L and free T$_4$ = 10.6 pmol/L.

N 27) A 30-year-old woman presents with heavy and painful periods of 12 months' duration. In addition, her periods are irregular varying from 4 weeks to 8 weeks. On examination, her BMI is 29 kg/m^2 and the uterus is normal in size. An ultrasound scan of the pelvis did not reveal any abnormality. Her hormone profile is as follows: prolactin = 732 mIU/L, FSH = 3.5 IU/L, LH = 7.4 IU/L, TSH = 2.6 IU/L, free T$_4$ = 12 pmol/L.

I 28) A 34-year-old female store supervisor presents with heavy periods of 2 years' duration. She has been treated by her GP with various drugs to no effect. Her periods are not painful and now last for 6 days instead of the usual 3–4 days. She has lost weight significantly over the last few months even through her appetite has paradoxically increased. Her tolerance to heat is rather poor. On examination, her BMI is 19 kg/m^2 and the pelvic organs are normal. Her hormone profile is as follows: prolactin = 346 IU/L, FSH = 6.6 IU/L, LH = 5.1 IU/L, TSH = 0.5 IU/L, free T$_4$ = 28 pmol/L.

29) A 30-year-old woman presents with heavy periods of 2 years' duration. She feels very weak by the end of each period and has been placed on iron tablets by her GP. On examination, her BMI is 24 kg/m^2 and the uterus is enlarged to the size of a 14-week pregnancy. It is irregular and firm in consistency. Her hormone profile is as follows: prolactin = 346 mIU/L, FSH = 2.6 IU/L, LH = 3.4 IU/L, TSH = 8.7 IU/L and free T$_4$ = 13 pmol/L.

Option list for Questions 30–31

A.	Amniotic fluid embolism
B.	Cardiac arrest
C.	Cord compression
D.	Cord prolapse
E.	Eclampsia
F.	Intracranial haemorrhage
G.	Placental abruption
H.	Postpartum haemorrhage
I.	Ruptured uterus
J.	Ruptured vasa praevia
K.	Shock – metabolic
L.	Shoulder dystocia
M.	Spinal block
N.	Supine hypotensive syndrome
O.	Thromboembolism
P.	Uterine inversion
Q.	Uterine atony
R.	Disseminated intravascular coagulation (DIC)

Instructions: The following pregnant women present with either fetal heart rate abnormalities or a complication of labour. Select from the option list above the **single** most appropriate cause of the heart rate abnormality or complication of labour. Each option may be selected once, more than once or not at all.

30) A 39-year-old gande multiparous woman in labour at 38 weeks' gestation presented with variable decelerations but good baseline variability. Fetal membranes are intact. A shift in the position improved the CTG.

A 31) A 39-year-old known gestational diabetic woman was induced because of her gestational diabetes and polyhydramnios. She started contracting 2 hours' after a 3 mg prostaglandin E_2 pessary. Three hours later she had an ARM. She progressed quickly to delivery (4 hours later) but soon after began to bleed easily from puncture sites. In addition, she also had tachypnoea and a low oxygen saturation rate in air.

Option list for Questions 32–33

A.	Aneuploidy
B.	Breast cancer
C.	Cancer in children
D.	Chromosome abnormalities
E.	Chronic myeloid leukaemia
F.	Ectopic pregnancy
G.	Endometrial cancer
H.	Growth discordancy in childhood
I.	Hyperemesis gravidarum
J.	Hypospadias
K.	Multiple pregnancies
L.	Ovarian carcinoma
M.	Ovarian cysts
N.	Ovarian hyperstimulation syndrome
O.	Preterm labour
P.	Prolonged hospitalization
Q.	Psychological distress
R.	Y chromosome deletion

Instructions: The couples below are undergoing ICSI as treatment for infertility. They have been given counselling about the risks of this procedure. Select from the above list of options the **single** most appropriate complication of ICSI that you would mention in relation to their concern. Each option may be selected once, more than once or not at all.

J 32) This couple were investigated for infertility and the man was found to be oligzoospermic while the women had blocked tubes and irregular ovulation. They were therefore offered ICSI with superovulation. They are anxious about malformations that may occur as a result of this procedure.

33) This couple have read several studies that have investigated the effect of ICSI on the offspring and are concerned about its subtle effects which do not manifest themselves as structural abnormalities.

Option list for Questions 34–37

A.	Acute intermittent porphyria
B.	Acute fatty liver of pregnancy
C.	Appendicitis
D.	Cholecystitis
E.	Constipation
F.	Diabetic ketoacidosis
G.	Domestic violence
H.	Ectopic pregnancy
I.	HELLP syndrome
J.	Hyperglycaemia
K.	Iliac vein thrombosis
L.	Labour
M.	Ligament pain
N.	Miscarriage
O.	Ovarian cyst – accident/haemorrhage/rupture
P.	Pancreatitis
Q.	Peptic ulcer
R.	Placental abruption
S.	Pneumonia
T.	Pre-eclampsia
U.	Pyelonephritis
V.	Renal colic
W.	Uterine fibroids

Instructions: For each of the following clinical scenarios, choose the **single** most likely cause of the abdominal pain from the option list above. Each option may be used once, more than once or not at all.

M 34) A 20-year-old woman presents at 18 weeks' gestation with bilateral sharp abdominal pain, which is occasionally like a stitch and aggravated by movement. The pain which started 2 weeks ago is shooting down her thighs. On examination, her pulse is 78 bpm, BP 118/66 mmHg, fundal height about 20 weeks, and the fetal heart is heard and is normal. Urinalysis is normal and her full blood count (FBC) is normal.

C 35) An 18-year-old primigravida presents at 29 weeks' gestation with a sudden onset of pain, which is mainly in the right lumbar region. The pain is associated with nausea and vomiting. Fetal movements are normal but she has not been able to open her bowels for the past 2 days. On examination, she is mildly pyrexial (temperature = 37.6°C), pulse 98 bpm and uterus about 30 cm. There is an area of marked tenderness over the right lumbar region with associated rebound. Her FBC shows mild leucocytosis and fetal CTG is excellent.

P 36) A 36-year-old G3P2 presents at 35 weeks' gestation with epigastric pain radiating to the back. The pain is accompanied by nausea and vomiting. On examination, her temperature is 37.1°C, pulse 94 bpm and fundal height 35 cm with a normal fetal heart rate. An ultrasound scan of the abdomen did not reveal anything abnormal but serum amylase is raised

Q 37) A 32-year-old primigravida presents at 32 weeks' gestation with pain which is mainly in the epigastric region. The pain radiates to the back and is aggravated by food. Much earlier, she had experienced heart burn and vomited blood once. On examination, her pulse is 82 bpm, BP 108/67 mmHg and the fundal height 33 cm with a normal CTG. Urine examination is normal.

Option list for Questions 38–40

A.	Achlorhydria test
B.	Blood film
C.	Bone marrow biopsy
D.	Red cell folate
E.	Chest
F.	Midstream urine specimen
G.	FBC
H.	Haemoglobin electrophoresis
I.	Liver function test
J.	Occult stool blood
K.	Protocolonoscopy
L.	Renal function test
M.	Serum B$_{12}$
N.	Serum ferritin
O.	Serum folate
P.	Stool examination

Instructions: For each of the clinical scenarios described below, choose from the option list above the **single** most useful investigation. Each option may be selected once, more than once or not at all.

38) A 33-year-old G6P5 is seen at the booking clinic when an Hb estimation was performed. A dating ultrasound scan showed a single fetus of appropriate gestation. Her Hb has been reported as 8.8 g/dL.

39) A 27-year-old woman presents with easy fatiguability after mild exertion and swollen feet at 28 weeks' gestation. She was found at booking to have an Hb of 10.5 g/dL. She was placed on iron tablets but failed to respond. She was then given parental iron but, once again, failed to respond. The blood film shows the following: mean corpuscular volume = 80 fL (80–99); mean corpuscular haemoglobin = 23.5 pg (27–32).

M 40) A 32-year-old woman presents for her routine antenatal care at 28 weeks' gestation when she is observed to be pale and tachycardic. She had her terminal ileum removed 3 years ago for complicated intussuception. The fundal height is compatible with her gestation.

3. Practice Paper 3: Answers

1) K.

IgM quantification in maternal blood and repeat if negative. This infection is likely to be parvovirus B19 and the presence of IgM in maternal blood will indicate infection. However, a negative test does not exclude the infection in the absence of symptoms. This should be repeated in 10–14 days.

2) P.

Cytomegalovirus can persist in the urine of infected babies for some years. A blood sample for antibodies is likely to be positive for IgG but this in itself does not necessarily mean that the baby was infected in utero.

3) B.

The most likely diagnosis is *Chlamydia trachomatis* and, for this, the best treatment option is azithromycin. It has the advantages that only a single dose is necessary and it is highly effective.

4) L.

The treatment for genital warts depends on the distribution of the warts. They are extensive and, therefore, excision is not the best option for this patient. Podophyllotoxin is effective provided that pregnancy has been excluded.

5) R.

The respiratory reserve of the patient will gauge the severity of her asthma. A respiratory peak flow volume will provide several indices of respiratory function including the respiratory reserve volume.

6) B.

The most likely diagnosis for this patient is pulmonary tuberculosis. The diagnostic tests for this include a Mantoux test, a chest X-ray, sputum for Ziehl–Neelsen stain and a bronchoscopy for PCR. PCR is the most reliable diagnostic test and is therefore the most appropriate option.

7) E.

Although she has been scheduled for surgery, staging is important in confirming that this is the correct procedure for her. An examination under anaesthesia (EUA), including cystoscopy, will help to clinically stage the disease and plan treatment. Although other investigations, such as a full blood count, urea and electrolytes, chest X-ray, and ultrasound scan of the abdomen are important and mandatory investigations, the one that is unique to this procedure is EUA.

8) **M**.
A mass of this size is likely to cause pressure effects on the ureter. Ultrasound scan of the abdomen will enable the ureter and kidneys to be examined for any pressure effects.

9) **P**.
This is an investigation that all women undergoing surgery for prolapse should undertake. For a woman with diabetes this is additionally important as any infections would be associated with significant postoperative morbidity.

10) **T**.
The options for this patient include: antibiotics, vaginal delivery or a caesarean section, steroids and amnioinfusion. There are features of chorioamnionitis and an irritable uterus. The baby needs delivering, but certainly not by elective caesarean section. Perhaps an emergency caesarean section would be an option, but this is not on the list of options. Delivery after antibiotics would, therefore, seem to be the most appropriate option. Amnioinfusion is contraindicated where there is chorioamnionitis.

11) **C**.
Since this patient has already had steroids, the most appropriate next step would be antibiotics – preferably erythromycin. There would be no need to deliver the baby until the features of chorioamnionitis are seen or the fetus is sufficiently mature to be delivered, e.g. after 34 weeks.

12) **O**.
This is already a high-risk pregnancy but is now complicated by reduced fetal movements. One of the fetuses is affected by an abnormality that is not compatible with life. The timing of delivery should be such that the normal fetus has the best chance of survival. The option that should be discussed with the patient is feticide of the abnormal fetus at the time of delivery and then delivery of both by caesarean section. This will remove the problems faced by a live baby with an abnormality that is not compatible with life. The ethics of this approach to the management of the patient must be discussed.

13) **N**.
Vulval ulcers associated with scarring are highly indicative of Crohn's disease.

14) **K**.
The characteristics of these lesions suggest a diagnosis of vulval Paget's disease.

15) G.

Sudden-onset chest pain in a 39 year old would suggest one of several possibilities: anxiety, aortic dissecting aneurysm, ischaemic heart disease, myocardiae infarction and pulmonary embolism. In this patient, the nature and location of the pain point to ischaemic heart disease.

16) C.

A dissecting aortic aneurysm is the obvious option for this patient, especially as she has a family history of Marfan's syndrome – a connective tissue disorder. Aortic regurgitation is a common finding in patients with Marfan's syndrome who are also likely to have aneurysms.

17) I.

The most likely diagnosis in this case is pneumonia because of the chest pain worsening on inspiration, the pyrexia and the leucocytosis. Although a pleural effusion will present in a similar way, this is less common than pneumonia.

18) J.

This is a classic presentation of tension pneumothorax caused by pushing in the second stage of labour. Although uncommon, it must be considered as a differential diagnosis in women presenting with unilateral chest pain following delivery.

19) J.

Features of Klinefelter's syndrome are typically tall, aggressive men who are infertile. They often have small testicles and a significantly abnormal semen analysis – the reason for their infertility. A differential diagnosis must include other causes of infertility where the men are tall and aggressive (although this may not be an inherited characteristic).

20) G.

The MAR test identifies the presence of antibodies that affect the fertilizing capacity of sperm. A positive MAR test in this patient would suggest the presence of sperm coated with antibodies which affects their fertilizing capacity.

21) H.

A combination of asthenozoospermia and chronic cough in this patient would suggest the immotile cilia syndrome. It is commonly seen in cystic fibrosis patients. However, it is not exclusive to cystic fibrosis as indicated by this patient who had no problems until 2 years before presenting with infertility.

22) K.

Transfer in utero is preferred to ex utero transfer in extremely premature babies. However, if delivery is considered to be imminent, then the former is considerably dangerous. In this case, although the cervix is 3 cm dilated, a combination of tocolysis and immediate transfer is most likely to be successful. A rescue cervical cerclage is unlikely to be successful. Steroids should be offered, but must be part of the package of in utero transfer. This comment also applies to atosiban.

23) N. ??
These twins exhibit growth discordancy and are likely to be affected by twin-to-twin transfusion. They require delivery and a middle cerebral artery Doppler will assist with the decision-making process. It is too late for laser division of the chorionic plate. Septotomy may be considered, but, if the babies are already affected at 32 weeks' gestation, delivery would be more beneficial than conservative management. In addition, if conservative management is to be undertaken it is important to ensure that neither of the fetuses is significantly compromised and requires immediate delivery.

24) T.
The surviving twin is recognized as being at risk of significant complications, the most severe of which involves the central nervous system. At 20 weeks' gestation, the surviving twin is already compromised and, therefore, the best option would be to offer a termination of the pregnancy.

25) M.
Features diagnostic of pelvic inflammatory disease in this patient include: the throbbing pelvic pain which worsens during menstruation, a fixed anteverted tender uterus and cervical motion tenderness.

26) G.
The clinical picture is that of a combination of irritable bowel syndrome and endometriosis – conditions that commonly coexist. The features of the enlarged ovaries are typical of endometriomas.

27) N.
Irregular periods, a high BMI and hyperprolactinaemia are suggestive of PCOS. Although the ratio LH:FSH is not typically high, it does not exclude PCOS.

28) I.
Hyperprolactinaemia can typically present with menorrhagia, increased appetite associated with weight loss and intolerance to heat. This patient's features suggest that the most likely diagnosis is hyperthyroidism. Her biochemistry confirms this diagnosis – low TSH and high free T_4.

29) O.
Uterine fibroids are the most obvious option for this patient. Although adenomyosis could be considered, the irregular nature of the uterus points to this differential diagnosis.

30) C.
The fact that the problem is eased with a change in the patient's position indicates that the most likely cause of a CTG abnormality is cord prolapse. Supine hypotension syndrome is another cause that can be rectified by changing the position of the patient. However, this commonly follows vaginal examinations with the patient in the dorsal position. In this case the patient presented with the deceleration and, therefore, cord compression is the most likely cause, especially as the fetal membranes were likely to be intact.

31) A.
Rapid progress, bleeding from puncture sites, tachypnoea and low oxygen saturation levels all point to amniotic fluid embolism. Pulmonary embolism is excluded because of the bleeding diathesis.

32) J.
The only structural abnormality that has been associated with ICSI is hypospadias in male fetuses.

33) R.
Deletions in Y chromosomes have been reported in babies delivered after ICSI, but the clinical relevance of these is uncertain.

34) M.
Ligament pain is common in pregnancy and typically presents with sharp lower abdominal pain which is aggravated on movement. The pain is often unilateral and improves with posture.

35) C.
The features of appendicitis in pregnancy are different from those seen in non-pregnant women. In this patient the diagnosis was based on systemic symptoms and localized tenderness lateral to the uterus on the right side.

36) P.
This is a very difficult diagnosis to be made but is based on a history of epigastric pain radiating to the back accompanied by nausea and vomiting. The investigations did not reveal anything abnormal except for a raised serum amylase level.

37) Q.
Peptic ulcer disease is rare in pregnancy but there may be significant consequences if the diagnosis is missed.

38) B.

A blood film will provide the most useful information about the type of anaemia involved. Only then can subsequent investigations be targeted at the different types of anaemia, i.e. iron deficiency or folate deficiency anaemia.

39) L.

The most likely cause of the non-refractory iron deficiency anaemia in this patient is renal dysfunction, possibly renal artery stenosis. In patients with renal dysfunction the production of erythropoietin is poor and they may fail to respond to iron even if given parenterally.

40) M.

The most likely cause of anaemia in this patient is a deficiency in vitamin B_{12} secondary to an inadequate absorption from the bowel as a result of the removal of the terminal ilium, which is the main site for the absorption of vitamin B_{12}. A serum vitamin B_{12} would, therefore, be the most informative investigation.

4. Practice Paper 4: Questions

Option list for Questions 1–4

A.	10
B.	80
C.	100
D.	150
E.	240
F.	270
G.	350
H.	420
I.	700
J.	800
K.	980
L.	1400
M.	1800
N.	2700
O.	96 000
P.	108 000
Q.	125 000
R.	139 000
S.	139 580
T.	140 000
U.	195 000
V.	210 000
W.	240 000

Instructions: Given below are figures for the births in a particular region. During a 1-year period, the stillbirth and perinatal mortality rates in the region were reported as 3/1000 and10/1000, respectively. There were a total of 420 stillbirths. From the information provided, select from the option list above the **single** correct number for each question.

1) What was the total number of births in the region? *T*

2) How many neonatal deaths occurred within the first week? *K*

3) What was the total number of perinatal deaths? *L*

4) What was the total number of live births in this region? *S*

Option list for Questions 5–7

A.	Air embolism
B.	Bladder damage
C.	Bowel obstruction from adhesions
D.	Damage to the pudendal nerve
E.	Detrusor overactivity
F.	Enterocele
G.	Pelvic abscess
H.	Perforation of the uterus
I.	Primary haemorrhage
J.	Residual ovary syndrome
K.	Stress urinary incontinence
L.	Subcutaneous emphysema
M.	Ureteric injury
N.	Urinary incontinence

Instructions: For each of following case scenarios, select from the option list above the **single** most likely and relevant short- or long-term complication that you will mention to the patient during preoperative counselling. Each complication may be selected once, more than once or not at all.

5) A 67-year-old woman, who had a total abdominal hysterectomy 8 years ago, presents with symptoms of vault prolapse and an associated rectocele and mild cystocele. She is scheduled to undergo an abdominal sacrocolpopexy.

6) A 48-year-old woman is scheduled to undergo an abdominal hysterectomy for menorrhagia and uterine fibroids. She is having her ovaries conserved as she is anxious about taking HRT and the associated risk of cardiovascular disease.

7) A 33-year-old woman presented with lower abdominal pain of 5 months' duration. On examination, she is found to have a large multiloculated mass arising from the pelvis. This is confirmed on ultrasound scan and is suggestive of a tubo-ovarian mass. Her CA-125 is 62 IU. She is scheduled for a laparotomy.

Option list for Questions 8–9

A.	*Actinomyces israelii*
B.	Bacterial vaginosis
C.	*Candida albicans*
D.	*Chlamydia trachomatis*
E.	Condylomata acuminata
F.	Dermatophytosis
G.	*Enterobius vermicularis* (threadworm)
H.	Filariasis
I.	Herpes simplex
J.	Human papillomavirus (HPV)
K.	Pediculosis
L.	Scabies
M.	Syphilis
N.	*Trichomonas vaginalis*
O.	Tuberculosis

Instructions: For each of the following, select from the option list above the **single** most likely cause of the vulval lesion. Each option may be selected once, more than once or not at all.

8) A 27-year-old woman who has just come from south-east Asia, presents with itching of the vulva which is worse at night and, occasionally, after a hot bath. She also has itching of her hands, armpits and buttocks. On examination, she is found to have a generalized papular rash of the vulva.

9) A 19-year-old woman, who has recently returned from a holiday
   in the Caribbean, presents with itching in the perianal and vulval
   areas of 3 weeks' duration. She has no vaginal discharge and
   sexual intercourse is not painful. Her last menstrual period was 2
   weeks ago. On examination, the only findings are multiple scratch
   marks on the vulva and perianal area.

Option list for Questions 10–12

A.	Aortic stenosis
B.	Cardiac hypertension
C.	Coarctation of the aorta
D.	Conn's syndrome
E.	Essential hypertension
F.	Flow murmur
G.	Mitral regurgitation
H.	Mitral valve prolapse
I.	Phaeochromocytoma
J.	Physiological
K.	Pre-eclampsia
L.	Pregnancy-induced hypertension
M.	Renal hypertension
N.	Tricuspid regurgitation
O.	Ventricular septal defect
P.	White coat hypertension

Instructions: For each of the following clinical scenarios, choose from
the option list above the **single** most likely cause of the murmur. Each
option may be used once, more than once or not at all.

10) A 19-year-old woman is seen in the antenatal clinic at 12 weeks'
    gestation for booking. On examination, she is found to have a very
    loud end-ejection systolic murmur associated with a palpable thrill,
    accompanied by an ejection click.

11) A 20-year-old primigravida presents for her booking visit and is
    found to have a BP of 150/94 mmHg. Urinalysis is normal. On
    auscultation of the heart, there is a systolic murmur but no other
    abnormality.

12) A 23-year-old primigravida attends for booking at 16 weeks' gestation. She is booking late as she is frightened of hospitals and has never been to see her GP. On examination, her BP is 150/96 mmHg. Her urinalysis is normal. There is a mild systolic murmur on auscultation.

Option list for Question 13

A.	Culture and sensitivity
B.	FSH
C.	Karyotype
D.	LH
E.	Mixed agglutination reaction (MAR) test
F.	Orchidometry
G.	Photomicrography
H.	Serum prolactin
I.	Semen analysis
J.	Sperm microscopy
K.	Testicular biopsy
L.	Testosterone
M.	Urethral swab
N.	Vasoepididymography
O.	Zona-free hamster oocyte test

Instructions: For each of the following cases, chose from the option list above the **single** most important investigation that you will perform on the patient in order to make a diagnosis of the cause of infertility. Each option may be selected once, more than once or not at all.

13) A 29 year old had a semen analysis for infertility. The results were as follows: count = 30×10^6/mL, motility = 60% with grade 3/4 motility and morphometry = 50% normal forms. There were 20 white cells present per high power field.

Option list for Questions 14–17

A.	Adrenal tumour
B.	Antidepressants
C.	Chronic renal failure
D.	Craniopharyngioma
E.	Cushing's syndrome
F.	Endometriosis
G.	Hypothyroidism
H.	Hyperprolactinaema
I.	Kallmann's syndrome
J.	Mumps oophoritis
K.	Pituitary tumour
L.	PCOS
M.	Premature menopause
N.	Prolactinoma
O.	Sheehan's syndrome
P.	Stress induced
Q.	Weight loss

Instructions: The following patients have been diagnosed with
anovulatory infertility. For each of them select from the option list
above the **single** most likely cause of the anovulation. Each option may
be selected once, more than once or not at all.

14) A 39-year-old woman presents with amenorrhoea and infertility. She
complains of an occasional discharge from her breast and loss of
libido. She was diagnosed as hypertensive 3 years ago and placed on
methyldopa which has controlled her blood pressure exceptionally
well. *H*

15) A 28-year-old woman presents with amenorrhoea and secondary
infertility. She delivered her only son 3 years ago. The pregnancy was
uncomplicated although she suffered from severe hypotension after
delivery. She was unable to breastfeed. *O*

16) A 22-year-old tall woman presents with primary amenorrhoea and
infertility. She has poorly developed secondary sexual characteristics
although her pubic and axillary hair are normal. She is sexually
active but is unable to distinguish coffee from tea.

17) A 30-year-old woman presents with amenorrhoea, headaches and intermittent vomiting. She has a whitish watery discharge from her breast but this is not constant. There is nothing abnormal found on examination. ⋈

Option list for Questions 18–20

A.	Acute cholecystitis
B.	Acute fatty liver of pregnancy
C.	Autoimmune chronic active hepatitis
D.	Coexisting liver disease
E.	Drug-induced hepatotoxicity
F.	Gallstones
G.	G6PD (glucose-6-phosphate dehydrogenase) deficiency
H.	HELLP syndrome
I.	Hyperemesis gravidarum
J.	Obstetric cholestasis
K.	Pre-eclampsia
L.	Pre-existing liver disease
M.	Primary biliary cirrhosis
N.	Sclerosing cholangitis
O.	Sepsis
P.	Thyrotoxicosis
Q.	Viral hepatitis

Instructions: For each of the following clinical scenarios, choose from the option list above the **single** most likely cause of the jaundice or the abnormal liver function test. Each option may be used once, more than once or not at all.

18) A 30-year-old primigravida at 27 weeks has been feeling generally unwell for the past week. There is associated nausea, anorexia and vomiting. Three days ago, she noticed that her eyes were yellow. On examination she is jaundiced and mildly tender in the right hypochondrion. Her liver function test shows raised bilirubin and moderate-to-severe elevation of transaminases.

19) A 27-year-old woman is admitted to the labour ward at 30 weeks' gestation with a 2-week history of nausea, anorexia, malaise, vomiting and abdominal pain. On examination, she is mildly jaundiced. Her BP is 140/90 mmHg and her urine has protein +.

Results of investigations undertaken show hyperuricaemia (very high), deranged liver enzymes and platelets of 80×10^9/L.

20) A 33-year-old G4P2 is admitted at 26 weeks' gestation with generalized malaise, nausea and vomiting of 1 week's duration. On examination, she is apyrexial, jaundiced and mildly anaemic. The fundal height is 24 cm and the fetal heart is heard and is normal. A liver function test shows a deranged liver function. She is positive for anti-smooth muscle antibody.

Option list for Questions 21–23

A.	Anastrazole
B.	Bromocriptine
C.	Cabergoline
D.	Clomifene citrate
E.	GnRH agonist and gonadotrophins
F.	Letrozole
G.	Metformin
H.	Motorized pulsatile GnRH agonists
I.	Ovarian drilling
J.	Pergonal (FSH and LH)
K.	Recombinant FSH
L.	Rosiglitazone
M.	Tamoxifen
N.	Trans-sphenoidal adenectomy
O.	Thyroxine
P.	Weight loss

Instructions: For each of the following patients presenting with infertility and anovulation, select from the option list above the **single** best method of induction of ovulation. Each option may be selected once, more than once or not at all.

21) A 29-year-old woman presents with primary infertility and amenorrhoea. Her BMI is 40 kg/m². The hormonal assays are as follows: FSH = 2.7 IU/L, LH = 12 IU/L, testosterone = 3.2 IU/L, sex hormone-binding globulin (SHBG) = 16, free androgen index (FAI) = 5%, prolactin = 765 mIU/L.

22) A 30-year-old woman presents with primary infertility and oligomenorrhoea. A postcoital test was negative when ovulation was achieved with clomifene citrate. An in-vitro sperm penetration test during one of the ovulatory cycles was negative. Her hormone profile is as follows: FSH = 6.7 IU/L, LH = 5.6 IU/L, prolactin = 236 mIU/L, testosterone = 0.6 IU/L, SHBG = 27, FAI = 54%.

23) A 30-year-old woman presents with primary infertility and irregular periods. Her BMI is 25 kg/m^2 and an ultrasound showed features consistent with PCOS. There was a suspicion of a tubo-ovarian mass on the right and she was therefore scheduled for a diagnostic laparoscopy. Her hormone assays were as follows: LH = 10 IU/L, FSH = 3.2 IU/L, testosterone = 3.6 IU/L, SHBG = 22 IU/L, FAI <7%, prolactin = 400 mIU/L.

Option list for Questions 24–26

A.	Amniocentesis for fluorescence in situ hybridization (FISH)
B.	Biophysical profile
C.	Chorionic villous sampling
D.	Fetal cardiac echo
E.	Fibrinogen
F.	Fibrinogen degradation products
G.	Genotype – fetal
H.	Karyotype for DiGeorge syndrome
I.	Kleihauer–Betke test
J.	Middle cerebral artery Doppler
K.	Nuchal translucency measurement
L.	Nuchal fold measurement
M.	Oral glucose tolerance test
N.	Platelet antibodies
O.	Pulmonary function test – L:S ratio
P.	Serum biochemistry at 15 weeks
Q.	Thrombophilia
R.	Umbilical artery Doppler
S.	Urea and electrolytes
T.	Uterine artery Doppler

Instructions: For each of the following clinical scenarios, choose from the option list above the **single** most aetiologically relevant factor or investigation. Each option may be selected once, more than once or not at all.

24) A 30-year-old woman is seen in the antenatal assessment unit of the hospital at 34 weeks' gestation with reduced fetal movements. She is sent for an ultrasound scan which reveals a cystic area in the fetal left cerebral hemisphere consistent with an intracranial bleed.

25) A 39-year-old woman presents with abdominal pain and vaginal bleeding at 30 weeks' gestation. This is her second pregnancy, the first having ended in an abruption and an intrauterine death. An ultrasound scan for growth shows that the baby is mildly growth restricted and there is a retroplacental haematoma measuring 6×8 cm. A CTG is normal.

26) A 30-year-old primigravida is seen at 20 weeks' gestation for her anomaly scan. She had an HbA1c of 9% (normal <6.1%) at booking (when she was at 10 weeks' gestation). The anomaly scan is normal.

Option list for Questions 27–29

A.	Adenomyosis
B.	Chronic renal failure
C.	Cushing's syndrome
D.	Dysfunctional uterine bleeding
E.	Endometrial hyperplasia
F.	Endometrial polyps
G.	Endometriosis
H.	Factor X deficiency
I.	Hyperthyroidism
J.	Hypothyroidism
K.	Idiopathic thrombocytopenic purpura (ITP)
L.	Intrauterine contraceptive device
M.	Irritable bowel syndrome
N.	Pelvic inflammatory disease
O.	PCOS
P.	Uterine fibroids
Q.	Von Willebrand's disease

Instructions: For each of the clinical scenarios presented below, choose from the option list above the **single** most likely cause of menstrual dysfunction. Each option may be selected once, more than once or not at all.

27) A 20-year-old woman presents with heavy and irregular periods. Her menarche was at 12 years of age and since then her periods have always been irregular. Although she suffers from acne, this is mainly during her periods. On examination, her BMI is 24 kg/m^2. Her pelvic organs are normal on ultrasound scan. Her hormone profile is as follows: prolactin 567 mIU/L, FSH = 4.6 IU/L, LH = 6.2 IU/L, TSH = 2.3 IU/L, free T$_4$ = 10 pmol/L and FAI = 5%.

28) A 27-year-old woman presents with secondary infertility and heavy and painful periods. She has been trying for a baby for the past 2 years without success. She experiences severe bloating of the abdomen just before and during menstruation. On examination, her BMI is 23 kg/m². The uterus is retroverted and slightly bulky. There is some induration of the uterosacral ligaments. Her hormone profile is as follows: prolactin = 267 mIU/L, FSH = 5.4 IU/L, LH = 4.7 IU/L, TSH = 1.2 IU/L and free T_4 = 12 pmol/L.

29) A 33-year-old woman presents with heavy and painful periods of 3 years' duration. The pains start a day before menstruation and persist for up to a few days after menstruation. She does not suffer from deep dyspareunia. Her GP has prescribed Cyklokapron to no effect. On examination, her BMI is 26 kg/m² and the uterus is uniformly bulky, to the size of an 8-week pregnancy. An ultrasound scan confirmed the bulky uterus but there were no obvious fibroids. Her hormone profile is as follows: prolactin = 600 mIU/L, FSH = 3.6 IU/L, LH = 4.3 IU/L, TSH = 2.7 IU/L, free T_4 = 12 pmol/L.

Option list for Questions 30–31

A.	Anuria
B.	Aplasia cutis
C.	Electrolyte derangement
D.	Fetal growth restriction
E.	Fluid retention
F.	Hyperglycaemia
G.	Hypokalaemia
H.	Hypotension
I.	Maternal tachycardia
J.	Pancytopenia
K.	Pancreatitis
L.	Pulmonary fibrosis
M.	Pulmonary oedema
N.	Renal failure
O.	Respiratory depression
P.	Angina
Q.	Pleurisy
R.	Hepatitis

Instructions: For each of the following clinical scenarios, choose from the option list above the **single** most likely complication of drug treatment for hypertension. Each option may be selected once, more than once or not at all.

30) A 28-year-old woman is admitted at 38 weeks' gestation with pre-eclampsia. Following prostin and ARM, she is commenced on oxytocin.

31) A 30-year-old known hypertensive woman books for antenatal care at 12 weeks' gestation. Her BP is 150/100 mmHg. She was placed on methyldopa which controlled her BP throughout pregnancy. She is now 36 weeks and complains of intermittent upper abdominal pains.

Option list for Questions 32–33

A.	Anxiolytics
B.	Bromocriptine
C.	Cabergoline
D.	Clomifene citrate
E.	Combined oral contraceptive pill
F.	Change medication from methyldopa to an ACE inhibitor
G.	Dialysis
H.	Discontinue medication
I.	Gonadotrophins
J.	In vitro fertilization
K.	Radiotherapy
L.	Reassurance
M.	Thyroxine
N.	Trans-sphenoidal adenectomy
O.	Weight gain
P.	Weight loss

Instructions: For each of the scenarios described below, select from the option list above the **single** most appropriate first-line treatment option for the patient's hyperprolactinaemia. Each option may be chosen once, more than once or not at all.

32) A 23-year-old female teacher presents with secondary amenorrhoea of 10 months' duration. She took up her new teaching appointment 12 months ago and is quite concerned about her ability to succeed as a teacher. Her BMI is 18 kg/m^2 and her prolactin is 805 mIU/L.

33) A 28-year-old woman attends with a milky discharge from her breast of 12 months' duration. Her periods are regular. She is currently using the combined oral contraceptive pill for contraception. On examination, her BMI is 32 kg/m^2. Prior to going on the pill, her periods were irregular. Her prolactin is 1045 mIU/L.

Option list for Questions 34–36

A.	Alcohol withdrawal
B.	Arteriovenous malformation
C.	Cerebral vein thrombosis
D.	Drug withdrawal
E.	Eclampsia
F.	Epilepsy
G.	Gestational epilepsy
H.	Hypoglycaemia
I.	Hypocalcaemia
J.	Hyponatraemia
K.	Idiopathic epilepsy
L.	Thrombotic thrombocytopenic purpura
M.	Ischaemic cerebral infarction or haemorrhagic stroke
N.	Postdural puncture
O.	Psuedoepilepsy
P.	Secondary epilepsy

Instructions: For each of the following clinical scenarios, choose from the option list above the **single** most likely cause of the patient's convulsions. Each option may be selected once, more than once or not at all.

34) A 30-year-old woman is admitted with prolonged and repeated seizures at 27 weeks' gestation. There is no history of previous fits. On examination, her BP is 130/88 mmHg, pulse 96 bpm; there is no cyanosis, the eyes are resistant to opening and the plantar reflexes are down-going. The conjunctival reflex is positive and persistent.

35) A 26-year-old woman is admitted into the labour ward at 33 weeks gestation with seizures. This is her first pregnancy and there is no prior history of seizures. On examination, her BP is 140/92 mmHg and reflexes are brisk. Urinalysis shows protein +++ and her FBC result is as follows: Hb 15.6 g/dL, platelets 89×10^9/L and WCC (white cell count) 8×10^9/L.

36) A 36-year-old woman who delivered 3 days ago following an induction of labour at 36 weeks' gestation for severe pre-eclampsia is re-admitted with convulsions. Analgesia during labour was by means of an epidural which also controlled the BP. There is associated neck stiffness, tinnitus and visual disturbances. Her BP is 150/92 mmHg and there is protein + in her urine. Her platelets are 150×10^9/L, WCC 12×10^9/L and Hb 12.4 g/dL.

Option list for Questions 37–38

A.	Basal body temperature
B.	Day 21 serum progesterone
C.	Endometrial biopsy
D.	Falloposcopy
E.	FSH and LH (serum)
F.	Hysteroscopy
G.	Hysterosalpingography
H.	Hysteroscopic contrast sonography (HyCoSy)
I.	In vitro mucus penetration test
J.	Laparoscopy and dye test
K.	Prolactin (serum)
L.	Postcoital test
M.	Salpingoscopy
N.	Spinnbarkeit
O.	Transvaginal ultrasound scan of the pelvis

Instructions: For each of the following case scenarios, select from the option list above the **single** most informative initial investigation that you will perform on the patient. Each investigation may be selected once, more than once or not at all.

37) A 26-year-old woman presents with infertility, headaches and an occasional discharge from the breast. She gives a history of having had a fracture to her skull 2 years ago.

38) A 26-year-old woman presents with primary infertility of 2 years' duration. She was investigated in her native country 2 years ago and had a dilatation and curettage. Since then her periods have become light, although they are still regular. Her husband's semen is normal.

Option list for Questions 39–40

A.	Anaemia
B.	Anxiety
C.	Drug induced
D.	Domestic violence
E.	Ectopic beats
F.	Hyperglycaemia
G.	Hypoglycaemia
H.	Physiological
I.	Severe asthma
J.	Sinus tachycardia
K.	Stress
L.	Supraventricular tachycardia
M.	Thyrotoxicosis
N.	Phaeochromocytoma

Instructions: For each of the following clinical scenarios, choose from the option list above the **single** most likely cause of the patient's palpitations. Each option may be used once, more than once or not at all.

39) A 21-year-old primigravida presents with palpitations which are intermittent and are worsen when the patient is lying in the supine position. The palpitations are associated with headaches, sweating and anxiety.

40) A 21-year-old female immigrant who does not speak English is admitted with palpitations of 3 weeks' duration. She has recently arrived in this country and is living with her husband's family. She has not yet reached 24 weeks' gestation. Nothing abnormal is found on examination.

4. Practice Paper 4: Answers

1) **T.**
140 000

2) **K.**
980

3) **L.**
1400

4) **S.**
139 580

The perinatal mortality rate is 10/1000. This is defined as the number of stillbirths and the number of neonatal deaths within 7 days of delivery over the total number of births. Since the stillbirth rate is 3/1000 and the total number of stillbirths was 420, the total number of births was therefore 140 000. The total number of perinatal deaths would have been 1400 and, when the stillbirths are subtracted from this, the total of early neonatal deaths would have been 980. The total number of live births was therefore 140 000 minus 420 giving a figure of 139 580.

5) **E.**
Long-term complications of sacrocolpopexy include urinary incontinence, enterocele, chronic backache and bowel obstruction including mesh erosion. In this scenario, although detrusor over-activity will present with urinary incontinence, it has other associated symptoms (such as frequency, urgency and nocturia) that are more specific.

6) **J.**
The long-term complications of the procedure include bowel obstruction from adhesions, enterocele and genital prolapse, residual ovary syndrome and urinary incontinence. However, urinary incontinence is not common and it is not a complication that it usually discussed with the patient. Residual ovary syndrome may, however, present with lower abdominal pain which may require surgery. It is, therefore, the complication that should be discussed in this case.

7) **C.**
Any surgery is associated with the risk of adhesion formation. This is greater for surgery performed on infected areas. The risk of adhesion formation in this patient with a probable tubo-ovarian abscess is considerably higher than after any other type of surgery. This complication should therefore be discussed with the patient.

8) L.

Itching of the vulva can be secondary to dermatophytosis, threadworms, pediculosis, scabies and warts. Itching which is worse at night is localized not only to the vulva but also to the armpits and buttocks, and is associated with a generalized papular rash typifying scabies.

9) G.

A history of holidays in the Caribbean and itching in the perianal area is highly suspicious of *Enterobius vermicularis* (threadworm). The scratch marks are of no significance as they are secondary to the scratching.

10) A.

A loud ejection systolic murmur with a palpable thrill accompanied by an ejection click is diagnostic of an aortic stenosis.

11) E.

The differential diagnoses here include essential hypertension, pre-eclampsia, renal hypertension, white coat hypertension and pregnancy-induced hypertension. Apart from essential hypertension, the others tend to be associated with other features or there are no murmurs. This is the case with white coat hypertension and pregnancy-induced hypertension.

12) P.

The fact that the patient has never been to the hospital and booked late suggests white coat hypertension.

13) A.

Further investigations could include a urethral swab, mixed agglutination reaction test, zona-free hamster oocyte test and sperm microscopy. The presence of 20 white cells per high power field suggests an infection and, for this, a culture and sensitivity of the semen would be the most important investigation.

14) H.

The amenorrhoea and infertility in this patient are most likely secondary to hyperprolactinaemia induced by methyldopa.

15) O.

Hypotension post delivery, followed by difficulties breastfeeding, amenorrhoea and infertility, is highly suggestive of Sheehan's syndrome.

16) I.

The classic clinical diagnostic feature of Kallmann's syndrome is the inability to distinguish between the smell of coffee and tea. Primary amenorrhoea as a presenting symptom should exclude all the causes of secondary amenorrhoea.

17) N.

The most likely cause of anovulation in this case is a pathology that causes headaches. A pituitary tumour, craniopharyngioma and prolactinoma are the three obvious options. A whitish discharge from the breast is indicative of hyperprolactinaemia, hence a prolactinoma is the most likely option.

18) Q.

There are several possible options for this question. However, the history of feeling unwell, and mild tenderness over the liver, make viral hepatitis the most likely choice. She is clinically not ill enough to have the other differentials such as acute fatty liver of pregnancy and HELLP syndrome.

19) B.

The main differential diagnoses here include HELLP syndrome, acute fatty liver of pregnancy and viral hepatitis. HELLP is unlikely because of her blood pressure, degree of proteinuria and biochemical abnormalities. Viral hepatitis will not present with such severely deranged liver enzymes. Therefore acute fatty liver of pregnancy is the most likely option.

20) C.

The positive anti-smooth muscle antibody is the main distinguishing factor in this case which leads to a diagnosis of autoimmune chronic active hepatitis.

21) P.

Although medical methods of induction of ovulation will suffice in this patient, the best option is weight loss. This offers several advantages over any of the medical methods. In addition, pregnancy is not advisable for women whose BMI is over 35 kg/m^2.

22) A.

Having failed to achieve a pregnancy with clomifene citrate, the best option will be a drug that will not affect the cervical mucus through its anti-estrogenic activities. Aromatase inhibitors have this advantage and hence this would be the best option for this patient.

23) I.

The patient is already scheduled for a diagnostic laparoscopy and so ovarian drilling would be the best option. Although the medical options will be equally effective, especially as she is not overweight, ovarian drilling has several advantages.

24) N.

Bleeding in the fetal brain may be caused by trauma, infection or neonatal alloimmune thrombocytopenia (NAIT). In this case, NAIT appears to be the most likely aetiological factor and can be diagnosed from platelet antibodies.

25) I.

The most likely cause of the fetal death is placental abruption. As there is likely to have been a significant fetomaternal haemorrhage, a Kleihauer test will be the best test option.

26) D.

This is an obviously diabetic mother whose fetus is at an increased risk of various malformations, including cardiac abnormalities. Since an anomaly scan at 20 weeks has already been described as normal, a fetal echo is essential because it may identify cardiac anomalies that were not identified at the anomaly scan.

27) D.

Anatomically and physiologically there is no obvious reason for the irregular bleeding. The most likely explanation for the menstrual disorders is, therefore, dysfunctional uterine bleeding.

28) G.

Options include adenomyosis, endometriosis, irritable bowel syndrome and pelvic inflammatory disease (PID). The history of pain starting before periods and persisting for days after is highly suggestive of endometriosis and adenomyosis. Although a bulky uterus on examination will support the diagnosis of adenomyosis, the bloatedness is more in keeping with endometriosis.

29) A.

The clinical picture is classic for adenomyosis, although endometriosis and PID should be considered in the differential diagnosis.

30) E.

Fluid retention is a complication of oxytocin infusion and this is seen more in women with pre-eclampsia.

31) K.

Intermittent upper abdominal pain could be secondary to the involvement of the cardiorespiratory and gastrointestinal systems. The most likely explanation in someone taking methyldopa is pancreatitis.

32) A.

The cause of this woman's hyperprolactinaemia is most likely to be anxiety and, therefore, anxiolytics should be the first option.

33) P.

There are two possible causes of the mild hyperprolactinaemia in this patient – drug induced (combined oral contraceptive pills) and due to her being overweight. Since there is no other option but for her to continue taking the contraceptive pill, the best option would be to advise her to lose weight.

34) O.
This is an unusual presentation. As it simulates epilepsy, the most likely cause of the convulsions is therefore pseudoepilepsy. There is no other option on the list to explain the clinical picture.

35) E.
The diagnosis in this case is very obvious, not only in view of the history, but also because of the biochemistry.

36) N.
Neck stiffness would immediately suggest meningitis. However, this is not associated with tinnitus and visual disturbances. Although she has pre-eclampsia, the features described do not support an eclamptic fit. The option that fits all these features is a postdural tap.

37) K.
A fracture to the base of the skull and a discharge from the breasts are likely to be related to hyperprolactinaemia, hence the best option will be serum prolactin.

38) G.
Hypomenorrhoea is the presenting feature for this patient following a dilatation and curettage. The most likely explanation for the hypomenorrhoea is Asherman's syndrome. This can be diagnosed by hysteroscopy or hysterosalpingography (HSG). Although the former allows diagnosis and treatment, the latter has the added benefit of enabling tubal patency to be assessed. Therefore, for this patient an HSG is the best option.

39) N.
The features point to a pathology that involves the production of sympathomimetics. A tumour is therefore the most likely cause of the symptoms.

40) K.
The absence of abnormality on examination suggests that the obvious explanation for the patient's symptoms is stress. This is supported by information about the patient's circumstances.

5. Practice Paper 5: Questions

Option list for Questions 1–4

A.	1:1
B.	1:2
C.	1:3
D.	1:4
E.	1:5
F.	1:10
G.	1:20
H.	1:25
I.	1:50
J.	1:75
K.	1:100
L.	1:150
M.	1:200
N.	1:250
O.	1:500
P.	1:750
Q.	1:1000
R.	1:1500
S.	1:2500
T.	1:5000
U.	1:7500
V.	1:10 000
W.	1:25 000
X.	1:50 000
Y.	No risk

Instructions: A couple attend for pre-pregnancy counselling about sickle cell disease. The genotype of the woman is HbAS and that of the husband is HbAC. For each of the questions raised by the couple below, select from the option list above the **single** most appropriate risk estimate that you will give them. Each option may be selected once, more than once or not at all.

1) What is the risk of the couple having a child with sickle HbSC disease?

2) What is the risk of their child being a carrier of the C genotype?

3) What is the risk of their child having a normal genotype?

4) If their daughter were a carrier and married a man with sickle cell anaemia, what would be the risk of their grandchild having sickle cell anaemia?

Option list for Questions 5–8

A.	Bowel injury
B.	Burst abdomen
C.	Damage to the iliac vessels
D.	Deep vein thrombosis
E.	Fluid overload
F.	Haematoma formation
G.	Infertility
H.	Incisional hernia
I.	Lymphocysts
J.	Paralytic ileus
K.	Pelvic abscess
L.	Rectovaginal fistula
M.	Richter's hernia
N.	Ureteric injury
O.	Ureteric ligation
P.	Vesicovaginal fistula
Q.	Wound infection

Instructions: For each of the following patients being counselled about gynaecological surgery, select from the option list above the **single** unique long-term complication associated with the surgical procedure. Each option may be selected once, more than once or not at all.

5) A 40-year-old woman undergoing balloon endometrial ablation for menorrhagia.

6) A 56-year-old obese woman undergoing a laparotomy for a large ovarian mass suspected to be a malignancy complicated by ascites.

7) A 26-year-old woman undergoing Wertheim's hysterectomy for carcinoma of the cervix stage Ia1.

8) A 30-year-old nulligravida woman who plans to have children undergoes a cold knife cone biopsy for CIN (cervical intraepithelial neoplasia) III and an incomplete colposcopy.

Option list for Questions 9–10

A.	Aciclovir
B.	Amitriptyline
C.	Azathioprine
D.	Benzyl benzoate
E.	Clotrimazole cream
F.	Cryotherapy
G.	Diathermy
H.	Excision
I.	Gabapentin
J.	Laser
K.	Marsupialization
L.	Mebendazole
M.	Metronidazole
N.	Podophyllotoxin
O.	Skinning vulvectomy
P.	Topical corticosteroids
Q.	Topical nystatin
R.	25% trichloroacetic acid

Instructions: For each of the following clinical cases, select from the option list above the **single** most appropriate first-line treatment option. Each option may be chosen once, more than once or not all.

9) A 27-year-old woman presented with widespread whitish lesions on the vulva associated with itching. Over the last 3 weeks these lesions have grown very rapidly and are becoming increasingly embarrassing. Her periods are generally irregular and the last one was 2 months ago. On examination, she is found to have widespread plaques covering most of the vulva. The largest measures approximately 2 mm in diameter.

10) A 30-year-old woman presents with a frothy green/creamy vaginal discharge. On examination, she is found to have an inflamed vulva and vagina. A high vagina swab demonstrates flagellates and clue cells.

Option list for Questions 11–13

A.	Atrioventricular malformation
B.	Cerebrovascular haemorrhage
C.	Cerebral vein thrombosis
D.	Cerebral ischaemia
E.	Drug-related headache
F.	Epidural-related headache
G.	Haemorrhage from aneurysm
H.	Hypertension/pre-eclampsia
I.	Idiopathic benign intracranial hypertension (pseudo-tumour cerebri)
J.	Meningitis
K.	Migraine
L.	Space-occupying lesion
M.	Spinal headache
N.	Subarachnoid haemorrhage
O.	Subdural haematoma
P.	Tension headache

Instructions: For each of the following clinical scenarios, choose from the option list above the **single** most likely cause of the headache. Each option may be used once, more than once or not at all

11) A 31-year-old obese G2P1 presents to triage with severe headaches at 20 weeks' gestation. She describes the headaches as being mainly behind the eyeballs, worse in the mornings and associated with double vision. On examination, her BP is 150/85 mmHg, urinalysis is negative for protein and there is bilateral papilloedema.

12) A 37-year-old primigravida is admitted with sudden and severe headaches which are mainly in the occipital region. There was associated vomiting at the outset. She collapsed before being brought into the hospital and, on examination, is found to have a temperature of 37.1°C, neck stiffness and focal neurological signs. Her BP is 130/76 mmHg and urinalysis is negative for protein.

13) A 34-year-old G3P2 presents at 32 weeks' gestation with severe headaches associated with seizures, vomiting, photophobia and impaired consciousness. On examination, there are features of hemiparesis, BP 133/88 mmHg and temperature 37.4°C. Her urinalysis is negative for protein. However, a white cell count shows leucocytosis.

Option list for Questions 14–15

A.	Combined oral contraceptive pill
B.	Danazol
C.	Depo-Provera
D.	Dimetriose
E.	GnRH agonist
F.	Hysterectomy
G.	Levonorgestrel intrauterine system (Mirena)
H.	Mefenamic acid
I.	Myomectomy
J.	Norethisterone
K.	Polypectomy
L.	Thermal balloon endometrial ablation
M.	Tranexamic acid
N.	Transcervical resection of the endometrium
O.	Uterine artery embolization

Instructions: For each of the following clinical scenarios, select the **single** most appropriate first-line treatment from the option list above. Each option may be chosen once, more than once or not at all.

14) A 44-year-old woman presents with a 4-year history of heavy periods that have failed to respond to medical treatment given by her GP. She has four children, one of whom requires constant care, and she is struggling to cope. She gets tired easily despite the iron tablets prescribed by her GP. She also suffers from depression. On examination, her BMI is 26 kg/m^2 and the size of her uterus is normal. Her Hb is 10.5 g/dL and a pelvic ultrasound is normal.

15) A 38-year-old Jehovah's witness, who was sterilized 6 years ago, presents with heavy periods of 5 years' duration. On examination she is found to have to a BMI of 29 kg/m^2 and a uterus enlarged to the size of an 18-week pregnancy. An ultrasound scan confirms that she has multiple fibroids. She was diagnosed to have a metabolic bone disease 4 years ago but cannot remember the exact type. Her Hb is 9.6 g/dL.

Option list for Question 16

A.	Amniocentesis for karyotype
B.	Amniocentesis for viral PCR
C.	Biophysical profile
D.	Cardiotocograph
E.	CT scan of the brain
F.	Detailed ultrasound scan
G.	Doppler of the middle cerebral artery
H.	Fetal blood sampling
I.	Fetal ECG
J.	Fetal haemoglobin electrophoresis
K.	Fetal blood group
L.	MRI of the brain
M.	Optical density of amniotic fluid
N.	Three-dimensional ultrasound scan
O.	Ultrasound scan
P.	Uterine artery Doppler
Q.	Fetal biometry measurement

Instructions: Select from the option list above the **single** most appropriate fetal investigation for the case scenario described below.

16) A 24-year-old primigravida attends the fetal assessment unit for fetal assessment at 28 weeks' gestation due to severe fetal growth restriction. The fundal height measures 24 cm and the amniotic fluid index is 5 cm (<5th centile for gestational age). The fetal heart rate auscultated with a Sonicaid is 168 bpm and is described as having unprovoked decelerations.

Option list for Questions 17–19

A.	Antibiotics
B.	Bowel anastomosis
C.	Cystoscopy
D.	Drainage
E.	Fistulogram
F.	Hysterectomy
G.	Immediate referral to gynaecological oncologist
H.	Immediate transfer to urology unit
I.	Indwelling catheter for 48 hours
J.	Indwelling catheter for 10 days
K.	Indwelling catheter for 10 days and antibiotics
L.	Instillation of alkylating agents in the peritoneal cavity and closure
M.	Laparotomy and repair
N.	Laparoscopic repair
O.	Lavage and drainage
P.	Nil by mouth for 48 hours
Q.	Observe for 24–48 hours
R.	Retrograde ureteroscopy
S.	Repair and colostomy
T.	Total abdominal hysterectomy, bilateral salpingo-oophorectomy and omentectomy
U.	Transfusion

Instructions: For each of the following case scenarios described below, select from the option list above the **single** most appropriate first-line management of the gynaecological surgical complication or findings. Each option may be selected once, more than once or not at all.

17) During laparoscopic adhesiolysis and resection of endometriosis, the left ureter of the patient is suspected of having been damaged by the laser during the dissection of the endometriosis over the ureter. There is no obvious evidence of leakage of urine from the site of the suspected injury.

18) A 30 year old is undergoing an ovarian cystectomy for a mucinous cystadenoma. At surgery, the cyst inadvertently ruptures and releases large quantities of viscid material into the peritoneal cavity.

19) During surgery for a suspected benign ovarian cyst, you discover that there are widespread metastases in the peritoneal cavity with ascites. There is a small ovarian cyst measuring 4 × 6 cm, with an irregular surface, and a capsule breached by tumour. You also suspect that the ureter is involved in the secondaries on the side wall.

Option list for Questions 20–21

A.	Adult respiratory distress syndrome
B.	Coagulation failure
C.	Cortical blindness
D.	Cortical renal failure
E.	Deep vein thrombosis
F.	Heart failure
G.	Hypoglycaemia
H.	Intracranial haemorrhage
I.	Liver failure
J.	Lupus nephritis
K.	Metabolic acidosis
L.	Myocardial infarction
M.	Pulmonary embolism
N.	Pyelonephritis
O.	Thrombocytopenia
P.	Thromboembolism
Q.	Wernicke's encephalopathy

Instructions: For each of the following case scenarios with medical complications of pregnancy described below choose the **single** important maternal complication from the option list above. Each option may be chosen once, more than once or not at all.

20) A 25-year-old woman, with a prosthetic heart valve for mitral stenosis, on heparin presented at 35 weeks' gestation in labour. The heparin levels were monitored with factor Xa levels antenatally. Shortly after delivery, she collapses and resuscitation is unsuccessful.

21) A 20-year-old primigravida presented with severe pruritus at week 32 of her pregnancy, and developed petechial haemorrhages 1 week after her admission for obstetric cholestasis and severe liver enzyme derangement. Following an induced vaginal delivery, she developed a massive postpartum haemorrhage from which she died.

Option list for Questions 22–25

A.	Brachytherapy
B.	Burns
C.	Carcinoma of the endometrium
D.	Colitis
E.	Combined external and intracavitary radiotherapy
F.	Cystitis
G.	Depression
H.	External radiation
I.	Intestinal obstruction
J.	Menopause
K.	Nausea and vomiting
L.	Point A
M.	Vaginal carcinoma
N.	Cervical stenosis
O.	Pyometria
P.	Fistula formation

Instructions: The following case scenarios refer to radiotherapy in gynaecological malignancies. Choose from the option list above the **single** most suitable applicable aspect of radiotherapy or its complication. Each option may be selected once, more than once or not at all.

22) A 28-year-old female teacher with stage IIa carcinoma of the cervix attends for radiotherapy and wishes to discuss the most severe complication that is likely to arise from the intracavitary source.

23) A 40-year-old woman underwent radiotherapy for carcinoma of the cervix. Two weeks later she presented with nausea and vomiting but no temperature.

24) A 31-year-old woman underwent Wertheim's hysterectomy for carcinoma of the cervix stage IIa. Histology of the removed pelvic organs shows carcinoma with involvement of the pelvic nodes.

25) A 33-year-old woman underwent radiotherapy for carcinoma of the cervix. She is now suffering from superficial dyspareunia, hot flushes and loss of libido.

Option list for Questions 26–28

A.	Absent or inappropriate ovaries
B.	Cervical mucus factor
C.	Endometriosis
D.	Failed artificial insemination with donor
E.	Failed ovulation induction
F.	Klinefelter's syndrome
G.	Male infertility
H.	Müllerian agenesis
I.	Pre-implantation diagnosis
J.	Premature menopause
K.	Therapy for female cancer
L.	Therapy for testicular cancer
M.	Tubal disease
N.	Turner's syndrome
O.	Unexplained infertility
P.	Cervical stenosis

Instructions: For each of the following patients undergoing assisted reproductive treatment (ART), select from the option list above the **single** most likely cause of the infertility. Each option may be selected once, more than once or not at all.

26) A 23-year-old woman presents with primary infertility. Her periods are regular and investigations of both partners revealed nothing abnormal. A postcoital test and a hamster egg penetration test are, however, abnormal.

27) A 22-year-old woman is undergoing ART after investigations for secondary infertility. She had a termination of pregnancy 2 years ago and, following that, suffered from abdominal pains and a foul smelling vaginal discharge, and was treated with antibiotics for 10 days.

28) A 30-year-old woman presents with secondary amenorrhoea and infertility. On examination, there is nothing abnormal. Her serum estradiol is 27 μmol/L, FSH is 34 IU/L and TSH is 20 IU/L.

Option list for Questions 29–30

A.	Antibiotics – intravenous
B.	Anticoagulation – full
C.	Elective caesarean section
D.	Emergency caesarean section
E.	Induction of labour
F.	Intramuscular opiates
G.	Intravenous fluids
H.	Intravenous fluids and thromboprophylaxis
I.	Intravenous fluids, antibiotics and thromboprophylaxis
J.	Lumbar epidural
K.	Middle cerebral artery Doppler
L.	Steroids
M.	Thrombolysis
N.	Thromboprophylaxis
O.	Transfusion with red cells
P.	Umbilical artery Doppler
Q.	Transfusion with whole blood

Instructions: For each of the following clinical scenarios choose from the option list above the **single** most appropriate intervention. Each intervention may be selected once, more than once or not at all.

29) A 27-year-old known HbSC presents at 32 weeks' gestation with intermittent mild abdominal pains which she has been having since 28 weeks. Her Hb is 8.7 g/dL and the fundal height is 29 cm. A CTG performed on admission is normal.

30) A 29-year-old G3P0 presents at 40 weeks with absent fetal movements for 24 hours. On examination, the fundal height is 40 cm, lie is longitudinal and the presentation is cephalic. The uterus is soft and the CTG shows a reduced baseline variability with neither accelerations nor decelerations after 40 minutes.

Option list for Questions 31–33

A.	Coitus interruptus
B.	Condom
C.	Copper multiload intrauterine device
D.	Diaphragm
E.	50 μg ethinylestradiol combined oral contraceptive pill
F.	Levonorgestrel intrauterine system (Mirena)
G.	Medroxyprogesterone acetate
H.	Mifepristone (RU486)
I.	Natural family planning
J.	Progestogen-only oral contraceptive pill
K.	Sequential combined oral contraceptive pill
L.	Sterilization – female
M.	Sterilization – male
N.	Subdermal implant (Implanon or Norplant)
O.	30 μg ethinylestradiol combined oral contraceptive pill
P.	Triphasic combined oral contraceptive pill
Q.	Levonelle 1500 μg stat
R.	Levonelle 750 μg stat
S.	Pregnancy test and copper IUD

Instructions: The patients below are attending for contraceptive advice. Select from the option list above the **single** most suitable form of contraception for the patient. Each option may be selected once, more than once or not at all.

31) A young woman attends the family planning clinic for contraception. She has had two terminations of unwanted pregnancies which have been secondary to missed oral contraceptive pills. She is in a steady relationship and her partner is considering using a barrier method.

32) A 20-year-old woman attends as an emergency having had unprotected sexual intercourse 3 days ago. She is quite anxious about an unwanted pregnancy.

33) A couple attend for counselling about contraception. They have completed their family and have so far been using the natural method of family planning. The woman is severely asthmatic and her BMI is 29 kg/m^2.

Option list for Questions 34–35

A.	Adrenarche
B.	Autoimmune hypothyroidism
C.	Congenital adrenal hyperplasia
D.	Constitutional
E.	Cushing's syndrome
F.	Ectopic gonadotrophin production
G.	Empty sella turcica syndrome
H.	Encephalitis
I.	Exogenous estrogen ingestion/administration
J.	Gonadotrophin-secreting tumour
K.	Harmatomas
L.	Hydrocephalus
M.	Irradiation
N.	Neurofibromatosis
O.	Ovarian tumour
P.	Polyostotic fibrous dysplasia (McCune–Albright syndrome)
Q.	Testicular tumour
R.	Third ventricle cyst

Instructions: For each of the following case scenarios select from the option list above the **single** most likely diagnosis. Each option may be selected once, more than once or not all.

34) An 8-year-old girl presents with well-developed breasts, pubic and axillary hair, and irregular menstruation of 4 months' duration. She

suffers from regular headaches which are relieved by paracetamol. On examination, she is found to have widespread café-au-lait spots of various sizes and shapes. Hormone profile is as follows: FSH <0.5 IU/L, LH <0.5 IU/L, 17β-estradiol = 260 mmol/L, prolactin = 670 mIU/L (50–400 mIU/L). An X-ray of the bone for maturity demonstrates multiple cystic lesions in the bones.

35) An 8-year-old girl presents with a regular menstruation of 7 months' duration and well-developed breasts, and pubic and axillary hair. She is overweight and complains of lack of energy. She has also noticed that, when she squeezes her breast, a whitish secretion comes out. On examination, she is 96.5 cm tall. Investigation results are as follows: X-ray of the skull shows enlarged sella turcica, TSH = 9 IU/L (0.3–4.0 IU/L), free T_4 = 8.9 pmol/L (15–25 IU/L), FSH = 6 IU/L, LH = 7.2 IU/L, 17β-estradiol = 217 mmol/L and prolactin = 850 mIU/L (50–400 mIU/L).

Option list for Questions 36–40

A.	Stage 1a G123
B.	Stage 1b G123
C.	Stage 1c G123
D.	Stage IIa G123
E.	Stage IIb G123
F.	Stage IIIa G123
G.	Stage IIIb G123
H.	Stage IIIc G123
I.	Stage IVa
J.	Stage IVb

Instructions: The following women have been diagnosed with a malignant disease of the uterus for which they have had surgery. Select from the option list above the **single** most appropriate stage of the malignancy. Each option may be selected once, more than once or not at all.

36) A 56-year-old woman presented with postmenopausal bleeding and had a hysteroscopy and endometrial biopsy that revealed poorly differentiated adenocarcinoma of the endometrium. She had a laparoscopically assisted vaginal hysterectomy and bilateral salpingo-oophorectomy. The histology report has revealed tumour invading to the serosa but there are no vaginal metastases.

37) A 49-year-old woman underwent a hysterectomy and bilateral salpingo-oophorectomy for atypical hyperplasia of the endometrium but the histology has been reported as carcinoma limited to the endometrium.

38) A 70-year-old woman receiving tamoxifen for breast cancer presented with postmenopausal bleeding of 6 months' duration. Following investigation, she had a hysterectomy and bilateral salpingo-oophorectomy. The histology showed cancer invading to the peritoneal surface with positive peritoneal cytology.

39) A 62 year old underwent surgery for carcinoma of the endometrium diagnosed from a pipelle endometrial biopsy. The histology report shows a well-differentiated carcinoma involving the endocervical glands but with invasion limited to less than 50% of the myometrium.

40) A 68-year-old diabetic woman presented with postmenopausal bleeding of 12 months' duration. She had an endometrial biopsy which was reported as a well-differentiated carcinoma of the endometrium. She has had surgery and, unfortunately, the histology report has come back indicating that the vagina has been invaded by the tumour.

5. Practice Paper 5: Answers

1) **D.**
   1:4

2) **D.**
   1:4

3) **D.**
   1:4

4) **B.**
   1:2

   Since both potential parents are carriers, the risk of any offspring having sickle cell HbSC disease will be 1:4. The risk of having a baby who will be a carrier is 1:4 for both HbAS and HbAC genotypes. The risk of having an unaffected child is 1:4. If their daughter was a carrier, and she married an affected male, then the risk of this couple having a grandchild with sickle cell disease will be 1:2.

5) **A.**
   The most common complications of balloon ablation of the endometrium are haemorrhage and secondary infections. Bowel injury is rare and often follows a perforation of the uterus.

6) **B.**
   A burst abdomen is a rare, but possible, complication following surgery in patients with an ovarian malignancy and ascites. This is more likely in a woman who is both obese and wasted.

7) **I.**
   Wertheim's hysterectomy can be complicated by haemorrhage, infections, injury to the urinary tract, especially the ureters, and adhesions followed by bowel obstruction. Lymphocysts are unique to this type of surgery and tend to be a long-term complication.

8) **G.**
   Removing the endocervix may result in cervical stenosis, dysmenorrhoea and haematocolpos if the cervix is completely stenosed. In pregnancy, it may result in mid-trimester miscarriages, preterm labour and dystocia in labour. However, the long-term gynaecological complication of infertility often results from removing the endocervix.

9) R.

The features are typical of condylomata acuminata which is best treated with 25% trichloroacetic acid.

10) M.

A greenish vaginal discharge which is associated with an inflamed vulva is most likely to be secondary to *Trichomonas vaginalis*. The presence of clue cells also suggests bacterial vaginosis. The treatment of choice for both conditions is metronidazole.

11) I.

Headaches, behind the eyes and worse in the morning, are highly indicative of benign intracranial hypertension. However, irrespective of other features, any hypertension in pregnancy warrants the exclusion of pre-eclampsia. In this patient, there is no proteinuria and bilateral papilloedema, which for mild hypertension is atypical of pre-eclampsia.

12) N.

Focal neurological signs and neck stiffness all point to an intracranial haemorrhage, although meningitis must be excluded. However, the absence of a temperature and severe headaches, predominantly in the occipital region, make this a less likely diagnosis.

13) C.

Although these features could be secondary to meningitis, the hemiparesis, impaired consciousness, seizures, vomiting and photophobia make a cerebral vein thrombosis more likely.

14) L.

An option that may be suitable for this patient is Mirena. However, as she has a child who requires constant care, she may struggle to cope with any irregular and unpredictable bleeding that may follow the use of Mirena. In addition, a hysterectomy will take her away from her child and will, therefore, be an unacceptable option.

15) O.

As this patient has completed her family a hysterectomy would be one of the best options. However, in view of her religion, she would not accept a blood transfusion and, therefore, the best option would be uterine artery embolization.

16) G.

Unprovoked decelerations occurring antenatally are difficult to interpret in isolation. In this patient the decision must be about immediate delivery or to continue to monitor and plan delivery, perhaps after steroids have been administered. A middle cerebral artery Doppler will identify those fetuses that require immediate delivery, although where reversal of compensation has occurred this may not be possible.

17) R.

The only way to confirm that the ureter has been damaged and to localize the site of injury is to undertake an imaging or endoscopic examination. The former would require the investigation to be undertaken while the patient was still under anaesthesia. The latter would easily be performed by a neurologist. The option of choice is, therefore, the one that is logistically easier to perform.

18) O.

In most cases, a lavage is adequate. However, this option is not given. Therefore, the only option closest would have to be lavage and drainage. Although the viscid material is known to cause pseudomyxoma peritonei, which can be fatal, there is no role for alkylating agents in its management or prevention.

19) G.

This patient clearly has what looks like an ovarian malignancy that has breached the capsule. Treatment will consist of a hysterectomy, bilateral salpingo-oophorectomy, omentectomy and chemotherapy after reviewing the histology. However, the immediate action must be to involve the oncologist who will then perform the surgery of choice.

20) M.

There are several risk factors for thrombosis in this patient and the most likely cause of her collapse is pulmonary embolism.

21) B.

She had features of either disseminated intravascular coagulation or coagulation failure.

22) P.

One of the most severe complications of radiotherapy in a young woman is radiation menopause. However, this is an acceptable consequence of the radiotherapy rather than an unexpected occurrence. The most severe complication which should be discussed with the patient is fistula formation – vesicovaginal or rectovaginal.

23) I.

The late presentation limits the differential diagnoses in this case. The symptoms of nausea and vomiting are all features of intestinal obstruction.

24) H.

Involvement of pelvic nodes suggests that surgical treatment is inadequate. Radiotherapy is therefore indicated.

25) J.

Superficial dyspareunia could be secondary to gynatresia induced by radiation burns. However, the association with hot flushes implies a more systemic side effect and radiation menopause would be the most likely cause.

26) B.

It is likely from the information provided that the cause of the infertility would be local at the level of the cervix, and this is therefore most likely to be secondary to excision of the endocervix with a resultant mucus factor abnormality.

27) M.

The most likely cause of the infertility in this young patient is tubal disease secondary to post-abortion infection. She developed abdominal pains and a foul smelling vaginal discharge after the termination of pregnancy.

28) J.

At this young age, the obvious explanation for the amenorrhoea and biochemical abnormalities is premature menopause. The precise reason for this is not clear from the information provided.

29) P.

Although she has intermittent mild abdominal pain, these have been occurring for more than 1 week. They are therefore likely to be Braxton Hicks' contractions. The fetus appears to be small and should be scanned but, since this is not an option, the next best option would be a Doppler of the umbilical artery. This will indicate just how compromised the fetus is if it is really growth restricted.

30) E.

This patient is term and has had reduced fetal movements for 24 hours. The fundal height is compatible with gestation and the cervix appears favourable for induction. There is no need for an emergency caesarean section but the fetus should be monitored continuously in labour.

31) N.

Having had two unwanted pregnancies on the combined oral contraceptive pill, this would not be a suitable method for this young girl. Although the partner is willing to use the barrier method, the condom would not be a very reliable method of contraception for her as its efficacy depends on the user who is not the patient. Subdermal implants will take away the problem of compliance and these are as effective as sterilization (female).

32) S.

Copper intrauterine device. Levonelle is effective if given within the first 72 hours. This patient has attended after 3 days and therefore this will no longer be highly effective. Although she gives a history of 3 days, a pregnancy test is crucial and she may well be pregnant.

33) M.
The woman is severely asthmatic and is slightly overweight. Since they have completed their family the man should be offered sterilization.

34) P.
The additional information on the X-rays of the bones makes the diagnosis easy.

35) B.
The most likely option here is autoimmune hypothyroidism on the basis of abnormal thyroid function test, short stature, obese and prolactinaemia.

36) F.
Stage IIIa G123 endometrial carcinoma.

37) A.
Stage Ia G123 endometrial carcinoma.

38) F.
Stage IIIa G123 endometrial carcinoma.

39) D.
Stage IIa G123 endometrial carcinoma.

40) G.
Stage IIIb G123 endometrial carcinoma.

Option list for Questions 1–3

A.	Central venous pressure
B.	Doppler of the fetal middle cerebral artery
C.	Elective caesarean section
D.	Emergency caesarean section
E.	Epidural analgesia
F.	Heparinization
G.	Intravenous opiates
H.	Intravenous fluids
I.	Intravenous antibiotics
J.	Intravenous Syntocinon
K.	Oxygen by facemask
L.	Prostaglandin E_2 pessary
M.	Re-examine in 4 hours
N.	Transfusion with whole blood
O.	Transfusion with packed cells
P.	Urgent ultrasound scan
Q.	Urgent full blood count

Instructions: For each of the following case scenarios choose from the option list above the **single** most appropriate management of the patient. Each option may be chosen once, more than once or not at all.

1) A 36-year-old woman with HbSC is admitted in labour at 38 weeks' gestation with irregular contractions which started 10 hours ago. The fetal membranes ruptured 2 hours after contractions began. The cervix was 4 cm on admission and her Hb was 8.1 g/dL.

2) A 20-year-old woman with HbSS presents with abdominal pain and dysuria at 33 weeks' gestation. On examination, she is mildly pyrexial, slightly dehydrated and pale. The fundal height is 30 cm

and the lie of the fetus is longitudinal. Urinalysis shows protein ++, nitrites ++ and blood +. Her Hb is 7.5 g/dL.

○ 3) A 27-year-old woman with HbSC, with a steady-state Hb of 8.9 g/dL, had a spontaneous vaginal delivery 2 hours ago. She is now complaining of breathlessness and palpitations. The estimated blood loss was 500 mL. On examination, she is pale, tachycardic (pulse = 126 bpm) and her blood pressure is 100/60 mmHg. The uterus is well contracted and her urine output is poor. Her Hb is 7.4 g/dL.

Option list for Questions 4–6

A.	Air embolism
B.	Bladder damage
C.	Bowel injury
D.	Bowel obstruction from adhesions
E.	Damage to the pudendal nerve
F.	Detrusor overactivity
G.	Enterocele
H.	Pelvic abscess
I.	Perforation of the uterus
J.	Persistent disease
K.	Primary haemorrhage
L.	Residual ovary syndrome
M.	Stress incontinence
N.	Subcutaneous emphysema
O.	Ureteric injury
P.	Urinary incontinence

Instructions: For each of following case scenarios, select from the option list above the **single** most likely and relevant short- or long-term complication that you will mention to the patient during preoperative counselling. Each complication may be selected once, more than once or not at all.

K 4) A 25-year-old woman presented with a 12-week amenorrhoea and excessive vomiting. An ultrasound scan showed an enlarged uterus containing a snow-storm appearance but no obvious fetal parts. She is scheduled for an evacuation of the uterus.

C 5) A 30-year-old woman had a subtotal abdominal hysterectomy for extensive endometriosis 4 years ago. She has now presented with recurrent deep pelvic pain and significant changes in bowel habits during menstruation. She is scheduled for a diagnostic laparoscopy.

G 6) A 48-year-old woman who presented with stress urinary incontinence underwent urodynamic investigations and was found to have urodynamic stress incontinence. She is scheduled to undergo Burch's colposuspension and is anxious about the long-term complications of the procedure.

Option list for Questions 7–10

A.	Cardiac malformations
B.	Chondrodysplasia punctata
C.	Duodenal hypertrophy
D.	Fetal growth restriction
E.	Heart block
F.	Intrauterine fetal death
G.	Macrosomia
H.	Meconium-stained liquor
I.	Necrotizing enterocolitis
J.	Neonatal hyperthyroidism
K.	Neonatal lupus
L.	Placental abruption
M.	Preterm labour
N.	Renal failure
O.	Spina bifida

Instructions: For each of the following case scenarios, choose from the option list above the **single** most likely/important/common fetal or neonatal complication of the maternal condition. Each option may be chosen once, more than once or not at all.

7) A 30-year-old primigravida, known to have Graves' disease, is seen at 36 weeks' gestation for routine antenatal care. She is on propylthiouracil which has controlled her thyrotoxicosis adequately.

8) A 31-year-old G2P0, who received a renal transplant 12 months ago, presents for booking at 12 weeks' gestation. She is on various antihypertensives and ciclosporin and her serum creatinine is >130 μmol/L.

9) A 34-year-old multigravida with epilepsy on lamotrigine attends the antenatal clinic at 12 weeks' gestation for booking. Her epilepsy is well controlled on this monotherapy.

10) A 32-year-old primigravida presents with polyhydramnios at 28 weeks' gestation which is treated with indometacin successfully.

Option list for Questions 11–12

A.	Antibiotics and repair 3 months later
B.	Boari's flap
C.	Conservative management (leave alone)
D.	Cystoscopy and repair
E.	Diagnostic laparoscopy
F.	Diuretics
G.	Drain the air with a Verres needle
H.	Immediate fistula repair
I.	Indwelling catheter and antibiotics for 10 days
J.	Repair alone
K.	Repair and colostomy
L.	Repair and lavage
M.	Repair and stent for 10 days
N.	Repair and indwelling catheter for 10 days
O.	Retrograde cystoureteroscopy
P.	Stop the procedure, antibiotics and observe for 24 hours
Q.	Ureteric implantation
R.	Ureteric stent

Instructions: The following complications were recognized at the time of surgery. Chose from the option list above the **single** most appropriate immediate step that you will take in dealing with the complication. Each option may be chosen once, more than once or not at all.

E 11) A 22-year-old woman presented with a 7-week amenorrhoea, vaginal bleeding and abdominal pains. On examination she is found to have an opened cervical os. A diagnosis of an incomplete miscarriage was made and she was offered an evacuation of retained products. During the procedure, the suction curette is found to pass effortlessly into the uterine cavity for almost the whole length of the cannula. She is, however, not bleeding.

L 12) A 22-year-old woman is undergoing laparoscopic surgery for endometriosis and a 0.5-cm-long small hole is found on the small bowel. This is most likely to have resulted from an accidental cut with laparoscopic scissors.

Option list for Questions 13–14

A.	Amniocentesis for chromosomes
B.	Amniocentesis for DNA
C.	Amniocentesis for OD 450
D.	Chorionic villous sampling for karyotype
E.	Chorionic villous sampling for DNA
F.	Coelocentesis
G.	Cervical flushing
H.	Fetal MRI
I.	DNA from clean voided specimen
J.	DNA from amniocentesis
K.	Low risk – hence reassurance
L.	Fetal blood sample (cordocentesis)
M.	Fetal DNA in maternal circulation
N.	Fetal cells in maternal circulation
O.	Maternal blood for DNA
P.	Paternal blood for DNA
Q.	Ultrasound scan

Instructions: The patients below presented for antenatal counselling about the risk of their baby having an inherited disorder. Select from the option list above list the **single** most appropriate piece of advice that you would offer the patient. Each option may be used once, more than once or not at all.

13) A 25-year-old woman, who is at 6 weeks' gestation in her first pregnancy, has a brother with cystic fibrosis (CF). Her partner is unrelated and has no family history of CF.

14) A 25-year-old woman, known to have HbAS, attends at 10 weeks' gestation for prenatal counselling about the risk of her baby having sickle cell disease. Her partner is HbAC.

A.	Abdominal hysterectomy and bilateral salpingo-oophorectomy
B.	Adhesiolysis
C.	Antibiotics – azithromycin
D.	Appendicectomy
E.	Combined oral contraceptive pill
F.	Diagnostic laparoscopy
G.	Endometrial ablation
H.	GnRH agonists
I.	Laser ablation of endometriosis
J.	Laparoscopic uterine nerve division (LUNA)
K.	Local injections with steroids
L.	Mefenamic acid
M.	Progestogen-only contraceptive
N.	Psychotherapy
O.	Steroid for inflammatory bowel disorder

Instructions: Choose the **single** most effective treatment that you will offer the patient from the option list above.

15) A 20-year-old woman presents with secondary dysmenorrhoea and severe abdominal pains which start with her periods and last until 2 days after her periods. She is not sexually active but has to use four superpads during menstruation.

Option list for Questions 16–17

A.	Acute pyelonephritis
B.	Aneurysm of the abdominal aorta
C.	Appendicitis
D.	Bowel obstruction
E.	Cholecystitis
F.	Diverticulitis
G.	Fitz–Hugh–Curtis syndrome
H.	Gallstones
I.	Hepatitis
J.	Intussusception
K.	Pancreatitis
L.	Pedunculated submucous fibroid
M.	Renal calculi
N.	Ruptured ectopic pregnancy
O.	Torsion of ovarian cyst

Instructions: All the women described below presented with acute abdominal pain. Select the **single** most likely cause of the acute pain from the option list above. Each option may be chosen once, more than once or not at all.

16) A 35-year-old woman presented with lower abdominal pains which are colicky in nature. Her periods have been heavy and associated with a dragging sensation for the past 6 months. On examination, she is pale. The uterus is approximately 10 weeks in size.

17) A 20-year-old woman presents with sudden-onset abdominal pain especially in the right hypochondrion. She is mildly pyrexial. On examination, she is tender in the right hypochondrion.

Option list for Questions 18–20

A.	Artificial sphincter
B.	Bladder overdistension
C.	Dopaminergic agents
D.	Duloxetine
E.	Flavoxate
F.	Glycinergic agents
G.	Imipramine
H.	Intravesical botulinum toxin injections (BTXa)
I.	Nervous GABA-ergic agents
J.	Oxybutynin hydrochloride
K.	Propantheline
L.	Propiverine
M.	Sacral nerve stimulation
N.	Solifenacin
O.	Tolterodine
P.	Trospium chloride
Q.	Vaginal estrogens

Instructions: For each of the patients presenting to the urodynamic clinic, select from the option list above the **single** most suitable first-line treatment for their urinary incontinence. Each option may be selected once, more than once or not at all.

18) A 56-year-old postmenopausal woman presents with stress urinary incontinence of 3 years' duration. She also suffers from nocturia, urgency and urge incontinence. Urodynamic studies were undertaken and she was found to have overactive bladder syndrome.

19) A 56-year-old postmenopausal woman presents with symptoms of nocturia, frequency and urgency. A urodynamic investigation was ordered and the results have come back indicating that she suffers from overactive bladder syndrome. She does not like taking tablets frequently.

20) A 56-year-old postmenopausal woman presents with symptoms of overactive bladder syndrome which is confirmed by urodynamic tests. She has had various treatments unsuccessfully.

Option list for Question 21

A.	Alcohol withdrawal
B.	Arteriovenous malformation
C.	Cerebral vein thrombosis
D.	Drug withdrawal
E.	Eclampsia
F.	Epilepsy
G.	Gestational epilepsy
H.	Hypoglycaemia
I.	Hypocalcaemia
J.	Hyponatraemia
K.	Idiopathic epilepsy
L.	Thrombotic thrombocytopenic purpura
M.	Ischaemic cerebral infarction or haemorrhagic stroke
N.	Postdural puncture
O.	Psuedo-epilepsy
P.	Secondary epilepsy

Instructions: Choose from the option list above the **single** most likely cause of the convulsions in the clinical scenario described below.

21) An 18-year-old primigravida is admitted with convulsions at 10 weeks' gestation. She had been complaining of excessive vomiting for the past week, and had been admitted and treated for 3 days before being discharged. Unfortunately, since arriving home she had failed to take her antiemetics for fear of teratogenicity. On examination, her BP is 100/55 mmHg and urinalysis: nitrites +, ketones +++ and protein +.

Option list for Questions 22–23

A.	Adrenal hyperplasia
B.	Anorexia nervosa
C.	Asherman's syndrome
D.	Bulimia
E.	Cervical mucus dysfunction
F.	Chlamydia salpingitis
G.	Cone biopsy
H.	Endometriosis
I.	Fetal bone
J.	Genital tract tuberculosis
K.	Hyperprolactinaemia
L.	Hypoplastic uterus
M.	Hypothyroidism
N.	Idiopathic
O.	Luteal phase defect
P.	Müllerian agenesis
Q.	Pituitary adenoma
R.	Polycystic ovary syndrome
S.	Sheehan's syndrome
T.	Stress induced

Instructions: For each of the following cases of infertility, select the **single** most probable cause of the infertility from the option list above. Each option may be selected once, more than once or not at all.

22) A 27-year-old woman presents with irregular periods, weight gain and primary infertility. On examination, she is found to have acanthosis nigricans and central adiposity.

23) A 32-year-old woman presents with secondary infertility of 3 years' duration. She had a cold knife cone biopsy for CIN III 4 years ago and, since then, has suffered from severe dysmenorrhoea. On examination, nothing abnormal is found.

Option list for Questions 24–26

A.	Age-specific mortality rate
B.	Crude mortality rate
C.	Early neonatal mortality rate
D.	Infant mortality rate
E.	Late neonatal death rate
F.	Maternal mortality rate (UK)
G.	Maternal mortality rate (WHO)
H.	Neonatal mortality rate
I.	Perinatal mortality rate (UK)
J.	Perinatal mortality rate (WHO)
K.	Standardized mortality ratio
L.	Stillbirth rate

Instructions: The following definitions are commonly used for statistical rates in reproductive medicine. For each definition, select from the option list above the **single** most appropriate rate referred to in the definition. Each option may be used once, more than once or not at all.

24) The total number of stillbirths after 24 weeks and neonatal deaths within 7 days of birth as a ratio to the total births per year.

25) The total number of deaths within the first 7 days of life, including live births before 24 weeks, as a ratio of all live births per year.

26) The ratio of observed deaths to expected deaths according to a specific health outcome in a population that serves as an indirect means of adjusting a rate.

A.	Interferon beta
B.	Chemotherapy
C.	Cone biopsy
D.	Cryotherapy
E.	Diathermy
F.	Excisional biopsy
G.	5-Fluorouracil
H.	Laser
I.	Levonorgestrel intrauterine system (LnG) (Mirena)
J.	Large loop excision of the transformation zone (LLETZ)
K.	Metronidazole
L.	Progestogens
M.	Radiotherapy
N.	Repeat colposcopy
O.	Simple vulvectomy
P.	Total abdominal hysterectomy
Q.	Total abdominal hysterectomy and bilateral salpingo-oophorectomy

Instructions: The following are descriptions of various pre-malignant gynaecological conditions. Choose from the option list above the **single** most suitable treatment for each scenario. Each option may be selected once, more than once or not at all.

27) A 36-year-old woman had an abnormal cervical smear for which a colposcopy was indicated. At colposcopy, the upper margin of the lesion could not be identified.

28) A 67-year-old woman presents with vulval itching of 12 months' duration. On examination, she is found to have multiple whitish plaques on both labia majora. There are no palpably enlarged inguinal nodes. A biopsy was performed and the histology is reported as hyperkeratinized squamous metaplasia consistent with VIN (vulval introepithelial neoplasia) III.

29) A 30-year-old woman presents with a vaginal discharge and soreness. She had a cervical smear which was reported as showing

severe dyskaryosis and *Trichomonas vaginalis*. A biopsy of the cervical lesion was reported as CIN III.

30) A 49-year-old morbidly obese woman (BMI 45 kg/m^2), presenting with irregular and heavy periods, had a hysteroscopy and biopsy as part of her investigation. The histology report shows that she has a complex hyperplasia without atypia.

Option list for Questions 31–32

A.	Assisted breech delivery
B.	Bakri balloon
C.	Brace suture
D.	Breech extraction
E.	Caesarean section
F.	Emergency caesarean section
G.	Fetal blood sampling
H.	Hysterectomy
I.	Internal podalic version and breech extraction
J.	Internal iliac artery ligation
K.	Intramuscular Syntometrine
L.	Intravenous ergometrine
M.	Kielland's forceps delivery
N.	Neville–Barnes forceps delivery
O.	Pack the uterus
P.	Recombinant factor VIIa
Q.	Uterine artery embolization
R.	Uterine artery ligation
S.	Transfusion with fresh whole blood
T.	Ventouse delivery with metal cup
U.	Ventouse delivery with Silastic cup
V.	Wrigley's forceps

Instructions: The following patients presented with postpartum haemorrhage. Choose from the option list above the **single** next most appropriate management for each patient. Each option may be selected once, more than once or not at all.

B 31) A 38-year-old primigravida who conceived twins after the fourth attempt at IVF was induced at 38 weeks' gestation. She had delivered the first twin 45 minutes ago. The membranes of the second twin are intact and the twin is lying longitudinally and presenting cephalic. Syntocinon was started 30 minutes ago and uterine contractions resumed shortly after. Soon after the second twin was delivered she developed severe postpartum haemorrhage which has failed to respond to all medications.

H 32) A 30-year-old primigravida had an emergency caesarean section 2 hours ago following an obstructed labour. She developed severe post-partum haemorrhage which has failed to respond to all forms of fertility-preserving treatment.

Option list for Questions 33–35

A.	Bilateral oophorectomy
B.	*Chlamydia trachomatis* treatment
C.	Combined oral contraceptive pill
D.	Condom
E.	Cytology
F.	Doppler of the pelvic arteries
G.	Endometrial biopsy
H.	Herpes simplex virus type 2 treatment
I.	Human immunodeficiency virus (HIV) treatment
J.	Human papillomavirus (HPV) treatment
K.	Hysteroscopy
L.	Magnetic resonance imaging
M.	Multiparity avoidance
N.	Cervical cytology
O.	Pelvic ultrasound scan
P.	Vaccination against HPV

Instructions: The patients described below are attending a gynaecology clinic for advice on the prevention of gynaecological malignancy to which they are at increased risk. Choose from the option list above the **single** most applicable method for each case. Each method may be chosen once, more than once or not at all.

D 33) A 28-year-old sex therapist presents with fears about carcinoma of the cervix. Her last cervical smear was 2 years ago and was normal.

C 34) A 30-year-old woman with a family history of ovarian cancer is quote anxious about the risk of developing ovarian cancer. Although there is nothing to suggest an ovarian malignancy, she would like to take preventive measures.

P 35) A 24-year-old woman presented with concerns about the risk of cervical cancer. She is in a steady relationship now, but is conscious of the fact that she has had many boyfriends in the past and is likely to have more in the future.

Option list for Questions 36–37

A.	Coincidental (fortuitous) maternal mortality
B.	Direct maternal death
C.	Early neonatal death
D.	Early neonatal mortality rate
E.	Early pregnancy death rate
F.	Indirect maternal mortality rate
G.	Infant mortality rate
H.	Intrapartum death
I.	Late fetal loss
J.	Late maternal mortality
K.	Late neonatal mortality
L.	Maternal mortality rate
M.	Neonatal mortality rate
N.	Perinatal morbidity
O.	Perinatal mortality rate (UK)
P.	Perinatal mortality (WHO)
Q.	Perioperative deaths
R.	Pregnancy-related death rate
S.	Stillbirth
T.	Stillbirth rate

Instructions: For each of the following descriptions, choose from the option list above the **single** most appropriate term. Each option may be used once, more than once or not at all.

L 36) The number of deaths from pregnancy, or within 42 days of the termination of pregnancy, from any cause related to or aggravated by the pregnancy or its management, but not from accidental or incidental causes, per 100 000 maternities.

37) Deaths resulting from a previous existing disease or disease that developed during pregnancy, which was not due to direct obstetric causes but which was aggravated by the physiological effects of pregnancy.

Option list for Questions 38–39

A.	Anterior repair
B.	Colposuspension
C.	Colpocleisis
D.	Diagnostic laparoscopy
E.	Hysteroscopy
F.	Manchester repair
G.	Myomectomy
H.	Ovarian cystectomy – laparoscopic
I.	Ovarian cystectomy – laparotomy
J.	Ovarian drilling
K.	Polypectomy
L.	Posterior repair
M.	Radiotherapy
N.	Sacrocolpopexy
O.	Sacrospinaous fixatioin
P.	Salpingectomy – laparoscopic
Q.	Subtotal hysterectomy
R.	Tension-free vaginal tape
S.	Total abdominal hysterectomy
T.	Total abdominal hysterectomy and bilateral salpingo-oophorectomy
U.	Trachelectomy
V.	Uterine artery embolization
W.	Vaginal hysterectomy
X.	Wertheim's hysterectomy

Instructions: For each of the case scenarios described below, choose the **single** most suitable surgical procedure from the option list above. Each option may be selected once, more than once or not at all.

38) A 30-year-old woman presents with lower abdominal pain, deep dyspareunia and heavy periods. On examination, she is found to be mildly pale but with a normal blood pressure and pulse rate. There are no abdominal masses. On pelvic examination, she is found to have an anteverted normal-sized uterus and bilateral adnexal tenderness. There is a palpable left adnexal mass measuring approximately 4 × 6 cm. It is doughy in consistency and appears to be attached to the uterus. The uterosacral ligaments are mildly indurated. An ovarian cyst is the provisional diagnosis.

39) A 40-year-old woman presenting with irregular periods of 6 months' duration is found, on examination, to have a bulky uterus which has descended to the level of the introitus. She underwent an endometrial biopsy and the histology report has come back with a diagnosis of hyperplasia with focal areas of atypia.

Option list for Question 40

A.	Amniotic fluid embolism
B.	Cerebral haemorrhage
C.	Cerebral infarction
D.	Cerebral vein thrombosis
E.	Eclampsia
F.	Hypoglycaemia
G.	Hypocalcaemia
H.	Hyponatraemia
I.	Placental abruption
J.	Pulmonary embolism
K.	Ruptured congenital aneurysm
L.	Ruptured uterus
M.	Seizures
N.	Subarachnoid haemorrhage
O.	Vasovagal attack
P.	Uterine hypotonia
Q.	Disseminated intravascular coagulation
R.	Spontaneous pneumothorax

Instructions: Select from the option list above the **single** most likely cause of collapse in the patient described below.

P 40) A 32-year-old G5P4 is admitted in spontaneous labour at 40 weeks' gestation. Fetal membranes are intact and the CTG is normal. She delivered after 1 hour's labour and has been bleeding profusely. During labour she complained of sharp pain in her chest and her abdomen but this was very short. Various attempts to stem the bleeding have failed and she has now collapsed.

6. Practice Paper 6: Answers

1) J.
The progress of labour in this high-risk patient has been slow and she would benefit from a Syntocinon augmentation of the labour.

2) I.
The clinical picture is consistent with that of urinary tract infection and immediate intravenous antibiotics would be recommended in order to minimize the rapid deterioration in her clinical state, including the development of sickle crises.

3) O.
Although the blood loss is only 500 mL, for someone whose steady-state Hb is only 8.9 g/dL, and who is now symptomatic, the best option would be transfusion with packed cells. Transfusion with whole blood should be avoided in these patients as the risk of overload is significantly greater.

4) K.
The complications of evacuating a molar pregnancy include primary haemorrhage, perforation of the uterus and persistent disease. Two of these are immediate complications; only persistent disease is a short- and long-term complication. However, the most likely complication is haemorrhage.

5) C.
The resulting adhesion formation following the patient's surgery will significantly increase the risk of bowel injury during the laparoscopy.

6) G.
Complications of this procedure, which is becoming increasingly less popular, include haemorrhage, injury to the bladder, difficulties in voiding after the surgery, detrusor overactivity and the development of an enterocele. As all the other complications are more common with this procedure, of which the patient is more likely to have been made aware, enterocele formation is the complication that should now be discussed.

7) D.
Thyrotoxicosis is associated with fetal growth restriction and preterm labour. At 36 weeks' gestation the fetal complication most associated with the condition is, therefore, fetal growth restriction.

8) D.

Although pre-eclampsia is one of the most common complications of renal transplantation in pregnancy, it is not a fetal complication. However, it may cause fetal growth restriction. Also note that fetal growth restriction may also caused by the drugs used to control hypertension.

9) D.

Well-controlled epilepsy is associated with an increased risk of congenital malformations, most of which depend on the antiepileptic medications being taken. In the absence of these malformations, as in this case, the risk of fetal growth restriction is greater than for those who don't have epilepsy.

10) N.

This drug is known to reduce renal perfusion and output; hence it is used in the treatment of polyhydramnios. However, renal failure is a well-recognized complication because of the effect on kidney perfusion.

11) E.

The suspicion here is that of uterine perforation. It is necessary to ascertain the extent of the injury to the uterus, whether it is bleeding actively (in which case it would require repair) or any viscera have been damaged. Although a diagnostic laparoscopy will not enable all of this to be achieved, it will support any subsequent evacuation from below.

12) L.

Any injury to the small bowel should be repaired at the time of surgery and adequate peritoneal lavage performed. There is usually no need for a colostomy or a drain to be left in situ.

13) O.

Since the brother of the woman has cystic fibrosis, the deletion responsible for this must be known. In the UK, the carrier rate for cystic fibrosis is approximately 1:22. However, not all the deletions are currently known. The first step would, therefore, be to determine whether or not the woman carries the same mutation as her brother. There will be no need at this stage to screen either the partner or the fetus.

14) E.

Both parents are carriers of the sickle cell trait. The risk of their baby having sickle cell HbSC is 1:4. They should, therefore, be offered testing in order to determine the genotype of the baby. At this early gestation this is commonly performed through chorionic villous sampling.

15) H.

The most likely cause of her symptoms is endometriosis. The gold standard treatment for this would be for the patient to be given the

GnRH agonist. If she were sexually active, it might have been better to start her on the combined oral contraceptive pill as GnRH agonists do not act as contraceptives.

16) L.

Heavy periods and a dragging abdominal pain suggest fibroid polyps. This is further supported by a 10-week-size uterus on examination.

17) G.

Abdominal pain associated with pyrexia in a young sexually active patient should raise the suspicion of infection with *Chlamydia trachomatis*. Localization of the pain in the right hypochondrion is pathognomonic of Fitz–Hugh–Curtis syndrome.

18) J.

The National Institute for Health and Clinical Excellence (NICE) recommends oxybutynin hydrochloride as the first-line treatment. It is also the most cost-effective.

19) N.

The NICE guidelines recommend solifenacin as an option for medical treatment of overactive bladder syndrome.

20) M.

Sacral nerve stimulation should be offered to patients with overactive bladder syndrome who have failed to respond to medical treatment.

21) J.

Although the urinalysis has generated features indicative of urinary tract infection, this is unlikely to be responsible for the fits. Since she had been vomiting excessively, the most likely complication presenting with these symptoms would be hyponatraemia.

22) R.

The presence of acanthosis nigricans will suggest either an adrenal problem or PCOS. In this case, she presented with weight gain, irregular periods and primary infertility which would make PCOS more likely.

23) E.

Removal of the cervical canal with a cone biopsy would have eliminated the secretions that, during ovulation, make the cervical mucus receptive to spermatozoa. She is likely to be suffering from cervical mucus dysfunction.

24) I.

Perinatal mortality (PNM), also perinatal death, refers to the death of a fetus or neonate and is the basis on which we calculate the perinatal mortality rate. Variations in the precise definition of the perinatal mortality exist which specifically concern the issue of inclusion or exclusion of early fetal and late neonatal fatalities. Thus, the World Health Organization's definition 'Deaths occurring during late pregnancy (at 22 completed weeks' gestation and over), during childbirth and up to seven completed days of life' is not universally accepted. The perinatal mortality is the sum of the fetal mortality and the neonatal mortality.

25) C.
Early neonatal mortality refers to a death of a live-born baby within the first 7 days of life. Late neonatal mortality covers the time after 7 days until 28 days. The sum of these two represents the neonatal mortality. Some definitions of the PNM include only the early neonatal mortality. Neonatal mortality is affected by the quality of in-hospital care for the neonate. Neonatal mortality and post-neonatal mortality (covering the remaining 11 months of the first year of life) are reflected in the infant mortality rate.

26) K.
The standardized mortality rate (SMR) is observed deaths $\times$ 100 expected deaths. The expected deaths are derived from the national figures, while the observed deaths reflect the real conditions. Thus, a comparison is made between national and local trends. An SMR of 100 indicates that the age-standardized mortality rate in the group being studied is the same as the overall, or standard, population. A ratio of less than 100 indicates a higher than average death rate; over 100 indicates a lower than average rate.

27) C.
This is an incomplete colposcopic examination and an indication for a cone biopsy.

28) O.
The absence of lymph nodes would be an indication for a simple excisional vulvectomy. In the past, radical vulvectomy used to the treatment of choice. However, the survival rate following radical surgery and simple vulvectomy has been shown to be same.

29) J.
The treatment of her incidental infection in not a priority, although she should be treated. The most appropriate treatment she should be offered is LLETZ.

30) I.
This is a morbidly obese woman who is obviously at risk of endometrial hyperplasia and cancer. She would be a major surgical risk and therefore conservative management would be most suitable. The LnG would be the treatment of choice.

31) B.

Once all the medical options have failed to control the haemorrhage, the surgical options should be considered. Delay in performing a hysterectomy has been blamed for some maternal deaths from massive postpartum haemorrhage. The first step should be to attempt a tamponade with a Bakri balloon, but this must be done in the theatre after having taken all the necessary precautions for a hysterectomy, or a Lynch suture if appropriate.

32) H.

For this patient, there is no place for further attempts to preserve the uterus. The best option is, therefore, a hysterectomy rather an embolization and internal iliac artery ligation.

33) D.

Barrier methods of contraception will reduce the transmission of the human papillomavirus which has been implicated in over 70% of cases of cervical cancer. The condom is, therefore, the most appropriate option.

34) C.

Although there are currently no know means of preventing ovarian cancer, the combined oral contraceptive pill is known to suppress ovarian activity and, thus, will reduce the risk of ovarian cancer.

35) P.

If the patient has not been exposed to the HPV antigen, vaccination would be an option for her. The current recommendations are to restrict vaccinations against HPV to adolescents.

36) L.

This is the definition of the maternal mortality rate.

37) F.

This is a description of indirect maternal deaths as detailed in the Confidential Enquiry into Maternal and Child Health (CEMACH) report.

38) D.

There is still some uncertainty about the findings in this patient. A diagnostic laparoscopy will assist the definition of the suspected clinical findings and the planning of further treatment, including surgery. Since any further surgery will be performed as an elective procedure, a diagnostic laparoscopy will provide information for the planning and discussions of alternatives with the patient.

39) W.

The treatment of choice for this woman is surgery. She already has a prolapsed uterus and, thus, a vaginal hysterectomy would be the most suitable approach to her hysterectomy.

40) P.

The potential causes of collapse in this patient include amniotic fluid embolism, cerebral haemorrhage, disseminated intravascular coagulation, pulmonary embolism and ruptured aneurysm. However, the history is not strongly supportive of any of these. She has been bleeding profusely after delivery. The most likely cause of the haemorrhage is hypovolaemia, rather than amniotic fluid embolism, as she does not have any respiratory symptoms. The chest and abdominal pain are detractors.

7. Practice Paper 7: Questions

Option list for Questions 1–4

A.	Box-and-whisker plots
B.	Between-subject variability
C.	Dot plots
D.	Histograms
E.	Fisher's exact test
F.	Interquartile ranges
G.	Negative predictive value of test
H.	95% confidence intervals
I.	Null hypothesis
J.	*P* value
K.	Pearson's correlation
L.	Positive predictive value of test
M.	Receiver operator curve
N.	Scatter plots
O.	Sensitivity
P.	Specificity
Q.	Standard deviation
R.	Student's *t*-test
S.	Survival curves
T.	Within-subject variability

Instructions: The following descriptions are for various statistical tools. Select from the option list above the **single** tool that best fits the description. Each option may be selected once, more than once or not at all.

1) A study was undertaken to determine the value of progesterone within a cohort of women presenting with secondary amenorrhoea. The data are presented as the difference between the upper and lower quartiles.

2) Joyce et al. (2009) undertook a study to measure the BP in 20 women prior to an elective hysterectomy following treatment of menorrhagia with the levonorgestrel intrauterine system. The data are presented as a box indicating the lower and upper quartiles and a central line representing the median.

3) Three hundred women with polycystic ovary syndrome and irregular periods underwent a screening test for endometrial cancer. Sixty per cent of the women with endometrial carcinoma are correctly identified by a positive test.

4) In the test above, 90% of those without endometrial carcinoma were correctly identified by the test.

Option list for Questions 5–8

A.	Adhesiolysis
B.	Aromatase inhibitor – anastrozole
C.	Bilateral salpingo-oophorectomy
D.	Combined oral contraceptive pill
E.	Danazol
F.	Depo-Provera
G.	Drainage of ovarian endometrioma
H.	Dydrogesterone (Duphaston)
I.	GnRH agonist
J.	Laser ablation
K.	Levonorgestrel intrauterine system (Mirena)
L.	Medroxyprogesterone acetate (Provera)
M.	Mefenamic acid (Ponstan Forte)
N.	Ovarian cystectomy
O.	Total abdominal hysterectomy
P.	Total abdominal hysterectomy and bilateral salpingo-oophorectomy
Q.	Tranexamic acid (Cyklokapron)

Instructions: For each of the following clinical scenarios, select from the option list above the **single** most effective first-line treatment that you will offer the patient. Each option may be selected once, more than once or not at all.

5) A 46-year-old woman presents with deep dyspareunia, dysmenorrhoea and severe premenstrual tension. On examination, she is found to have a retroverted bulky uterus and bilateral ovarian masses which, after an ultrasound scan, were confirmed to be ovarian endometriomas.

6) A 30-year-old nulliparous woman presents with deep dyspareunia and menorrhagia. On examination, she is found to have nothing abnormal. A diagnostic laparoscopy revealed widespread endometriosis (mainly powder-burn spots) in the pouch of Douglas and adhesions between the bowel and the pelvic side wall. The GP has tried simple medical treatment unsuccessfully.

7) A 34-year-old woman presents with menorrhagia and abdominal bloatedness. She is not on any form of contraception and has no need for any. A diagnostic laparoscopy revealed mild endometriosis.

8) A 37-year-old woman presents with lower abdominal pain and heavy periods which are not painful. An ultrasound scan has shown the presence of bilateral ovarian cysts measuring 6×8 cm and 8×9 cm. The features of the cysts are consistent with endometriomas. Her CA-125 is 50 iu. At diagnostic laparoscopy the findings are confirmed.

Option list for Questions 9–10

A.	Bell's palsy (facial nerve palsy)
B.	Carpal tunnel syndrome
C.	Diabetes mellitus
D.	Epidural block
E.	Guillain–Barré syndrome
F.	Hyperventilation
G.	Lumbosacral trunk
H.	Meralgia paraesthetica (lateral cutaneous nerve of the thigh)
I.	Migraine
J.	Multiple sclerosis
K.	Transient ischaemic attacks
L.	Vitamin B_{12} deficiency

Instructions: For each of the following clinical scenarios, choose from the option list above the **single** most likely cause of the numbness. Each option may be used once, more than once or not at all.

9) A 20-year-old woman presented to her GP at 20 weeks' gestation complaining of numbness, weakness and a tingling sensation in her legs. This has been progressively getting worse and is beginning to affect her upper limbs. On examination, there is motor weakness on the lower limbs with minimal weakness of the upper limb muscles. Her BP is 130/68 mmHg and the fundal height is 22 cm.

10) A 29-year-old primigravida is seen as an emergency at 39 weeks' gestation complaining of right facial weakness and an inability to wrinkle her forehead on the right side. She has pain around the ear and is unable to taste with the front of her tongue. On examination, her BP is 150/95 mmHg and her uterine fundus measured 40 cm.

Option list for Questions 11–13

A.	Clotting screen
B.	Colposcopy
C.	Diagnostic laparoscopy
D.	Examination under anaesthesia
E.	Full blood count
F.	Group and cross-match/save
G.	Hysteroscopy
H.	Intravenous urogram
I.	Liver function test
J.	Magnetic resonance imaging
K.	Pipelle endometrial biopsy
L.	Thyroid function test
M.	Triple swabs
N.	Ultrasound scan of the abdomen and pelvis
O.	Ultrasound scan of the pelvis
P.	Urea and electrolytes

Instructions: For each of the following case histories choose from the option list above the **single** most important investigation that you will undertake. Each option may be selected once, more than once or not at all.

11) A 34-year-old woman presents with superficial and deep dyspareunia of 3 years' duration. In addition, she complains of difficulties emptying her rectum during menstruation. A pelvic examination revealed a fixed retroverted bulky uterus with possible adnexal masses and an induration over the uterosacral ligaments, with a suspicion of bowel involvement in the disease.

12) A 30-year-old woman presents with a 9-months history of intermittent menstrual bleeding. Her periods are otherwise regular. She has had two pregnancies, all delivered at full term. On examination, she is found to have a normal-size anterverted uterus and nothing else abnormal.

13) A 37-year-old African–Caribbean woman presents with very heavy and painful periods of 5 years' duration. At the end of each period she feels weak and listless. Her last period which has just ended lasted for 14 days. On examination, she is found to have a 24-week-sized multiple fibroid uterus.

A.	Admit for emergency surgery
B.	Arrange an examination under anaesthesia
C.	Arrange urgent anaesthetic review
D.	Cancel surgery
E.	Cancel surgery and arrange an MRI
F.	Cancel surgery for today, rebook and offer appropriate treatment
G.	Cancel surgery and arrange further investigations
H.	Defer surgery for 1 month
I.	Defer surgery for 3 months
J.	Discharge from the specialty
K.	Discuss an alternative procedure and proceed after counselling
L.	List for diagnostic laparoscopy and dye test as a routine procedure
M.	List for diagnostic laparoscopy and dye test as a soon procedure
N.	List for laparoscopy and diathermy
O.	List for surgery and to have bowel preparation
P.	List for surgery to be performed within 2 weeks
Q.	List for surgery to be performed within 2 months
R.	Place on the waiting list for a diagnostic laparoscopy
S.	Postpone surgery and arrange an MRI/further investigations
T.	Proceed with surgery as planned
U.	Refer for surgical opinion before placing on the waiting list
V.	Review results of investigations and proceed with surgery

Instructions: The following patients are on the waiting list for surgery, need to be placed on the waiting list or have attended for surgery. Some of the procedures have been listed properly or need to be listed while others need change or modification. Review each case and select from the option list above the **single** most appropriate step for the patient. Each option may be selected once, more than once or not at all.

14) A 56-year-old woman was seen in the gynaecology clinic 4 days ago with a pelvic mass that was suspected to be an ovarian malignancy. She had a liver function test, urea and electrolytes, a full blood count

and CA-125. The CA-125 was 230 iu (markedly raised) and she was placed on the list for surgery to be performed 2 days later. She is now attending the preoperative clinic to discuss surgery.

15) A 16-year-old girl is admitted for termination of pregnancy at 12 weeks' gestation. She is found to be pyrexial and urinalysis has revealed nitrites and proteinuria. She feels achy and generally very queasy

16) A 27-year-old woman is scheduled for a diagnostic laparoscopy and dye test as part of investigations for infertility. She attends for this procedure and reveals that she has broken up with her partner and is now in a new relationship.

17) A 60-year-old woman attends for planned surgery for a pelvic mass which was suspected to be a benign ovarian cyst. She had an MRI of the abdomen and pelvis and a CA-125. The results are not in her notes.

18) A 42-year-old woman has been admitted for Wertheim's hysterectomy. She complains of an offensive vaginal discharge and lower abdominal pain.

19) A 50-year-old obese woman has been listed for Burch's colposuspension because of urodynamic urinary stress incontinence. She has a mild asymptomatic cystocele.

Option list for Questions 20–21

A.	Atosiban
B.	Azathioprine
C.	Augmentin
D.	Beta-sympathomimetics
E.	Carbamazepine
F.	Carbimazole
G.	Corticosteroids
H.	Diet control
I.	Digoxin
J.	Erythromycin
K.	Free thyroxine (FT$_4$)
L.	Insulin
M.	Metformin
N.	Propranolol
O.	Propylthiouracil

Instructions: For each of the case scenarios described below, choose the **single** most suitable first-line treatment (prophylactic or therapeutic) from the option list above. Each option may be chosen once, more than once or not at all.

20) A 30-year-old woman presents at 30 weeks' gestation with preterm prelabour rupture of fetal membranes which occurred 3 hours previously. On examination, she is apyrexial and the abdomen is non-tender, symphysial fundal height measures 27 cm with cephalic presentation and a normal CTG. A speculum examination confirms rupture of fetal membranes.

21) A 29-year-old primigravida presents at 35 weeks' gestation with preterm prelabour rupture of the fetal membranes which occurred an hour before presentation. On examination, she is found to have a mildly tender abdomen but the fetal CTG is normal. Rupture of fetal membranes is confirmed by speculum examination.

Option list for Questions 22–23

A.	Bucket-handle
B.	Circumferential
C.	Cruciate
D.	Grid-iron (over McBurney's point)
E.	Hunter's point
F.	Infraumbilical transverse
G.	Infraumbilical vertical
H.	Lower transverse with division of recti muscles
I.	Midline subumbilical
J.	Palmer's point
K.	Paramedian – longitudinal
L.	Pfannenstiel
M.	Posterior fornix transverse
N.	Posterior fornix midline
O.	Suprapubic transverse
P.	U-shaped

Instructions: The following patients are on the waiting list for surgery. Choose from the option list above the **single** most suitable incision for the surgical procedure offered. Each option may be chosen once, more than once or not at all.

22) A 50-year-old woman presents with an abdominal mass, poor appetite and dyspepsia. On examination, she is found to have an irregular abdominal mass which appears to be separate from the uterus. There is associated ascites. An ultrasound scan shows an irregular, partly solid and partly cystic mass arising from the left ovary. The ascites is confirmed. She is scheduled for surgery by the gynaecological oncologist.

23) A 26-year-old woman, who presented with three episodes of post-coital bleeding, underwent a colposcopically directed biopsy. The report has come back as invasive carcinoma of the cervix. After examination under anaesthesia the disease is classified as stage Ia. She is scheduled for Wertheim's hysterectomy.

Option list for Questions 24–26

A.	Acute cholecystitis
B.	Acute fatty liver of pregnancy
C.	Autoimmune chronic active hepatitis
D.	Coexisting liver disease
E.	Drug-induced hepatotoxicity
F.	Gallstones
G.	G6PD deficiency
H.	HELLP syndrome
I.	Hyperemesis gravidarum
J.	Obstetric cholestasis
K.	Pre-eclampsia
L.	Pre-existing liver disease
M.	Primary biliary cirrhosis
N.	Sclerosing cholangitis
O.	Sepsis
P.	Thyrotoxicosis
Q.	Viral hepatitis

Instructions: For each of the following clinical scenarios, choose from the option list above the **single** most likely cause of the jaundice or abnormal liver function test. Each option may be used once, more than once or not at all.

24) A 33-year-old G4P2 is admitted at 26 weeks' gestation with generalized malaise, nausea and vomiting of 1 week's duration. On examination, she is apyrexial, jaundiced and mildly anaemic. The fundal height is 24 cm and the fetal heart is heard and is normal. A liver function test shows a deranged liver function. She is positive for anti-smooth muscle antibody.

25) A 26-year-old female teacher is admitted at 33 weeks into her first pregnancy complaining of generalized itching, which she has had for a few years, and jaundice, which was noticed only a few weeks ago. On examination, she is moderately jaundiced and her liver is enlarged. A liver function test shows a markedly elevated alkaline phosphatase but nothing else abnormal. She is anti-mitochondrial antibody positive.

26) A 30-year-old female typist, who is known to have Crohn's disease, presents at 32 weeks' gestation with intermittent pruritus which has recently been accompanied by jaundice. Investigation results show evidence of chronic inflammation.

Option list for Question 27

A.	Adoption
B.	Bromocriptine
C.	Follicle-stimulating hormone (FSH)
D.	Gamete intrafallopian transfer (GIFT)
E.	In vitro fertilization and embryo transfer (IVE-ET)
F.	Intracytoplasmic sperm injection (ICSI)
G.	Intrauterine insemination with donor sperm
H.	Intrauterine insemination with husband's sperm
I.	Orchidopexy
J.	Percutaneous sperm aspiration and ICSI
K.	Reassurance
L.	Salpingotomy
M.	Sperm washing and insemination
N.	Steroids for antisperm antibodies
O.	Testosterone injections
P.	Varicolectomy
Q.	Vitamin E

Instructions: Select from the above list of options the **single** most appropriate initial treatment option for this couple with infertility.

27) A couple attend the gynaecology outpatient department with secondary infertility. Investigations reveal that the woman was ovulating normally and also had patent fallopian tubes. However, on examination, the man was found to have obstructive azoospermia.

Option list for Questions 28–29

A.	Anaemia
B.	Aortic stenosis
C.	Arrhythmias
D.	Cerebral oedema
E.	Drug induced
F.	Exhaustion
G.	Fluid overload
H.	Hyperglycaemia
I.	Hyperpyrexia
J.	Hypertrophic cardiomyopathy
K.	Hypoglycaemia
L.	Hypothyroidism
M.	Idiopathic hypotension
N.	Labyrinthitis
O.	Massive haemorrhage
P.	Postural hypotension
Q.	Sepsis
R.	Supine hypotension syndrome

Instructions: For each of the following clinical scenarios, choose from the option list above the **single** most likely cause of the dizziness. Each option may be used once, more than once or not at all.

28) A 19-year-old woman is seen in the antenatal clinic at 28 weeks when she complained of frequent dizzy spells which have got worse as her pregnancy has advanced. She also suffers from palpitations. Her tolerance to exercise is poor as she becomes easily breathless on mild exertion. On examination, her BP is 132/77 mmHg, urinalysis is negative, and her pulse is described as irregular and 120 bpm.

29) A 20-year-old woman presents with breathlessness, chest pain and dizzy spells at 32 weeks' gestation. On examination, her BP is 120/77 mmHg, urinalysis is negative, there is a double apical pulsation (palpable fourth heart sound) and a pansystolic murmur.

Option list for Questions 30–34

A.	CIN I
B.	CIN II
C.	CIN III
D.	Stage O
E.	Stage Ia1
F.	Stage Ia2
G.	Stage Ib1
H.	Stage 1b
I.	Stage Ib2
J.	Stage IIa
K.	Stage IIb
L.	Stage IIIa
M.	Stage IIIb
N.	Stage IVa
O.	Stage IVb

Instructions: The following women have been diagnosed with either a premalignant or a malignant disease of the cervix. They have, however, not been staged. Select from the option list above the **single** most appropriate stage of the malignancy. Each option may be selected once, more than once or not at all.

30) A 32-year-old woman presented with postcoital bleeding of 2 months' duration. She was found to have a suspicious lesion on the anterior lip of the cervix. This was biopsied and was, subsequently, reported as squamous cell carcinoma. She had an ultrasound of the abdomen and there was bilateral hydronephrosis. On examination, under anaesthesia, the disease was thought to be limited to the parametrium but the side wall was not involved.

31) An examination under anaesthesia was performed on a 41-year-old woman with carcinoma of the cervix. A cystoscopy revealed bullous oedema of the bladder with no obvious lesions. The parametrium was involved up to the side wall.

32) A 39-year-old woman was diagnosed with carcinoma of the cervix after a routine abnormal cervical smear. She underwent an examination under anaesthesia and the tumour was confined to the cervix. A chest X-ray and an ultrasound scan of the abdomen were all normal.

33) A 51-year-old woman, who has recently been diagnosed with carcinoma of the cervix, was found to have a tumour extending to the lower third of the vagina and oedema of the bladder on cystoscopy. The parametrium was involved but not to the side wall. Her abdominal ultrasound scan and chest X-ray were both normal.

34) A 26-year-old woman attended for colposcopy following an abnormal cervical smear. Macroscopically there were no suspicious areas, but a biopsy obtained showed a squamous carcinoma of the cervix with a 4-mm depth of stromal invasion.

Option list for Question 35

A.	Computed tomography scan of the brain
B.	Dehydroandrosterone sulphate (DHEAS)
C.	Dexamethasone suppression test
D.	Free androgen index (FAI)
E.	Serum calcium
F.	Serum FSH and LH
G.	Serum prolactin
H.	Serum testosterone
I.	Short Synacthen test
J.	Thyroid function test
K.	Thyroid peroxidase antibody
L.	24-hour cortisol measurement
M.	Ultrasound scan of the abdomen
N.	Ultrasound scan of the pelvic organs
O.	Urinary hydroxysteroids
P.	Urinary vanillylmandelic acid (VMA)

Instructions: Select from the option list above the **single** most informative investigation that you will recommend for the following patient.

35) A 17-year-old woman presents with hirsutism shortly after puberty. She states that her older sister had a similar problem. Her periods have also become irregular but her weight has not increased significantly. She has become darker in her axilla. Her serum testosterone, measured by her GP, is reported as 6 nmol/L (normal 1–4).

Option list for Questions 36–40

A.	Addison's disease
B.	Adrenal insufficiency
C.	Anaemia
D.	Conn's disease
E.	Cushing' syndrome
F.	Diabetes mellitus pre-gestational
G.	Gestational diabetes
H.	Hyperprolactinaemia
I.	Hypothyroidism
J.	Panhypopituitarism
K.	Phaeochromocytoma
L.	Pituitary insufficiency
M.	Postpartum thyroiditis
N.	Primary aldosteronism
O.	Prolactin-producing adenomas
P.	Thyrotoxicosis
Q.	Type 1 diabetes mellitus

Instructions: For each of the clinical scenarios described below choose from the option list above the **single** most appropriate diagnosis. Each option may be selected once, more than once or not at all.

36) A previously healthy 35-year-old woman delivers a 4.2 kg baby at 38 weeks after an induction of labour for reduced fetal movements and a non-reassuring cardiotocograph. In the latter stage of her pregnancy, she complained of increasing frequency of micturition and recurrent vulvovaginal abscesses.

37) A 27-year-old woman delivers a macrosomic male baby at 38 weeks' gestation following induction of labour for polyhydramnios. The baby is found to have a congenital malformation and is unable to control his body temperature.

38) A 19-year-old woman undergoes an induction of labour for fetal growth restriction and absent umbilical artery Doppler at 36 weeks' gestation. During pregnancy, she complained of palpitations and intermittent diarrhoea.

39) A 30-year-old woman delivers a baby at term that is found to be floppy and slightly growth restricted. During pregnancy she suffered from listlessness, poor tolerance to cold and general lack of energy.

40) A 30-year-old mother of three, on large doses of steroids for severe asthma presents in labour. Her previous labour was precipitate. Thirty minutes after presentation, she had a spontaneous vaginal delivery and lost about 700 mL of blood. The uterus is now well contracted but she has suddenly collapsed (BP 80/50 mmHg, pulse 90 bpm) with a weak volume.

7. Practice Paper 7: Answers

1) F.

One way in which data are presented is in quartiles. The 25th and the 75th centiles are known as quartiles and these values, together with the median, divide the data into four equally populated subgroups. The numerical difference between the 25th and the 75th centiles is the interquartile range.

2) A.

A box-and-whisker plot is a box showing the upper and lower quartiles and the central line represents the median. The points at the ends of the whiskers are 2.5% and 97.5% values.

3) O.

Sensitivity is the proportion of positives that are correctly identified by a test. This is also occasionally referred to as true positives.

4) P.

Specificity is the proportion of negatives that are correctly identified by the test. This is occasionally referred to as true negatives.

5) P.

It is most likely that this patient has adenomyosis and bilateral endometriomas. Medical treatment in the form of a GnRH agonist will not be suitable for the endometriomas. Although the sizes of endometriomas are not given, surgery would be the most appropriate option. In view of her age, and the severe premenstrual tension, this would ideally be a hysterectomy and bilateral salpingo-oophorectomy.

6) I.

The best option to start with is a GnRH agonist which is considered as the gold standard medical treatment option. This is unlikely to have been tried by the GP.

7) D.

Her symptoms are most likely secondary to endometriosis and, therefore, medical treatment would be the first option. Her abdominal bloatedness, though possibly related to her endometriosis, may also be linked to ovulation. Suppressing ovulation and, at the same time, offering treatment for endometriosis would seem the logical approach to her management and, as such, the combined oral contraceptive pill should be considered the first option.

8) N.
The endometriomas in this patient measure more than 5 cm and would, therefore, require surgery. Drainage is not the recommended treatment. Ovarian cystectomy is, therefore, the treatment of choice.

9) E.
This is an uncommon presentation in obstetrics, but the progressive nature of the clinical presentation and associated motor weakness on the lower limbs are features of Guillain–Barré syndrome.

10) A.
This is a classic presentation of Bell's palsy.

11) J.
A diagnostic laparoscopy will confirm endometriosis, which is the most likely diagnosis. However, it will not diagnose adenomyosis and bowel involvement. An MRI is, therefore, the most important investigation.

12) G.
An important differential diagnosis in this patient is endometrial polyps (possibly small fibroids) which are causing the intermittent menstrual bleeding. A hysteroscopy would be the best option for making a diagnosis. Although an ultrasound scan of the pelvis will identify polyps and fibroids, the gold standard diagnostic investigation is a hysteroscopy.

13) E.
Investigations that this patient should be offered include an ultrasound scan of the abdomen and pelvis, urea and electrolytes and blood group testing (especially if she will require surgery or transfusion). However, in view of her history, the most urgent investigation has to be a full blood count as she may well be so anaemic as to require blood transfusion.

14) S.
This patient has an obvious ovarian malignancy which has not been properly staged. She requires investigations to exclude secondaries in the liver and chest and to note the extent of the spread within the abdomen. It is important to perform a chest X-ray and abdominal MRI/CT scan before proceeding to surgery. This will enable better planning for the surgery and counselling.

15) F.
This procedure is scheduled to be performed under general anaesthesia. If she has a respiratory tract infection, this may be associated with significant morbidity. It is, therefore, advisable to postpone the surgery and offer more appropriate treatment which may include antibiotics and analgesics.

16) **G**.

Before a woman being investigated for infertility is subjected to any invasive procedure, it must be certain that there is no male factor involved. In this case, there is no evidence that she has tried having a baby long enough with her current partner. While she may find the cancellation of the surgery upsetting, it would be inappropriate to undertake this procedure without ensuring that the new partner wants to have children with her, that they have been trying for the required length of time and that his semen is normal.

17) **V**.

The results of the investigations should be reviewed and, if normal, the surgery should then be undertaken. This is important because a raised CA-125 is suspicious of an ovarian malignancy the treatment of which is likely to be different from that of a simple ovarian cyst.

18) **T**.

This woman has cervical cancer and an offensive vaginal discharge is a recognized presentation of cervical malignancy. There is, therefore, no need to postpone her surgery.

19) **K**.

Surgical treatment for urodynamic stress incontinence is currently Burch's colposuspension or tapes that can be offered in different ways. This patient is obese and her main symptom is stress urinary incontinence. It appears that, so far, only Burch's colposuspension has been discussed. The tape procedures should now be discussed and the option that she chooses offered if the expertise is available.

20) **G**.

Preterm delivery and chorioamnionitis are the two complications of prelabour preterm rupture of fetal membranes. The administration of corticosteroids and antibiotics will minimize these complications. However, steroids should be the first option as they are most effective if given at least 24–48 hours before delivery.

21) **J**.

At this gestation, respiratory distress syndrome is not a major consequence of delivery. However, infections remain an important complication and, hence, antibiotics should be administered. Erythromycin is the antibiotic of choice.

22) **K**.

The clinical features are highly indicative of an ovarian malignancy and surgery for this patient should be via a paramedian or midline incision. The risk of a burst abdomen and an incisional hernia is greater with a midline incision. A paramedian is therefore preferred.

23) H.
Wertheim's hysterectomy can be performed through a midline, paramedian or pfannenstiel (lower transverse) incision with the division of the rectus muscles. The last option is the most cosmetically acceptable and achieves the same degree of access as a vertical incision.

24) C.
A positive anti-smooth muscle antibody and features of systemic illness are highly indicative of autoimmune chronic hepatitis.

25) M.
The absence of systemic symptoms and a positive anti-mitochondrial antibody is indicative of primary biliary cirrhosis.

26) N.
Sclerosing cholangitis is the most obvious option in view of the intermittent pruritus, Crohn's disease and features of inflammation.

27) J.
Options include adoption, ICSI, intrauterine insemination with donor sperm and percutaneous sperm aspiration. The last option is the most suitable as the man has obstructive azoospermia which implies that he does produce sperms that can be aspirated and used in vitro.

28) C.
An irregular pulse associated with dizzy spells, poor tolerance to exercise and palpitations are all indicative of arrhythmias.

29) J.
The typical feature of hypertrophic cardiomyopathy on clinical examination is a palpable fourth heart sound and a pansystolic murmur.

Note: Questions 30–34 refer to the different stages of carcinoma of the cervix. The answers to these questions are quite straightforward provided that the candidates understand the staging of this common malignancy.

30) M.
Although an examination did not demonstrate a spread to the parametrium, the presence of hydronephrosis will indicate that this has indeed happened. An examination under anaesthesia will not reliably define the extent of the spread to the side wall. The stage of this disease is, therefore, IIIb.

31) M.

Here the tumour has extended to the side wall and there is bullous oedema of the bladder. Bullous oedema of the bladder is not considered as bladder involvement in the staging of carcinoma of the cervix, hence the stage remains IIIb.

32) G.

The patient has macroscopic disease which is confined to the cervix, hence it is stage Ib.

33) L.

The parametrium is involved but it has not extended to the side wall. The lower third of the vaginal is involved, implying that the cancer is stage IIIa.

34) F.

This is microscopic disease diagnosed from a biopsy at colposcopy. The depth of invasion is less than 5 mm and, hence, the cancer is stage Ia2.

35) I.

The patient most probably has Cushing's syndrome and a short Synacthen test will be the most useful investigation to undertake.

36) F.

Recurrent vulvovaginal abscesses and a macrosomic baby at 38 weeks' gestation are features of diabetes mellitus.

37) F.

Congenital malformations are not recognized features of gestational diabetes. This woman must have had pre-existing diabetes which was poorly controlled during pregnancy.

38) P.

Thyrotoxicosis is the most likely diagnosis in this patient because of the growth restriction, palpitations and intermittent diarrhoea.

39) I.

The possible options include Cushing's syndrome, hypothyroidism, Addison's disease and anaemia. Poor tolerance to heat, lack of energy during pregnancy and a floppy, mildly growth-restricted baby would be highly suggestive of hypothyroidism.

40) B.

The features reflect a poor response to the stress of labour which is common in cases of adrenal insufficiency.

Option list for Questions 1–6

A.	45 XO
B.	45 XO/46 XY
C.	45 XX, rob(14;21)(q10q10)
D.	45 XY, rob(13;21)(q10q10)
E.	46 XX
F.	46 XX, add(20)(p13)
G.	46 XX, del(14)(p13)
H.	46 XX, del(18)(q21)
I.	46 XX, der(2)t(2;12)(p14;p13)
J.	46 XX, r(15)
K.	46 XX, t(2;12)(p14;p13)
L.	46 XY
M.	46 XY, der(2)t(2;12)(p14;p13)
N.	46 XY, fra(X)(q27.3)
O.	46 XY, inv(5)(p14;q15)
P.	46 XY, t(2;12)(p14;p13)
Q.	47 XX + 13
R.	47 XX + 18
S.	47 XX + 21
T.	47 XXY
U.	47 XY + 13
V.	47 XY + 18
W.	47 XY + 21
X.	47 XYY
Y.	69 XXX
Z.	69 XXY

Instructions: For each of the following cases choose from the option list above the **single** most appropriate description of the chromosome abnormality obtained from karyotyping for prenatal diagnosis. Each option may be chosen once, more than once or not at all.

1) A 38-year-old primigravida booked for antenatal care at 10 weeks' gestation. She requested a nuchal translucency test which came back with a risk of 1:150. She opted for a chorionic villous sampling (CVS) and fluorescence in situ hybridization (FISH) indicated that the female fetus had Patau's syndrome.

2) A 16-year-old girl presents with primary amenorrhoea and failure to undergo adrenarche. On examination, she is found to have a heart murmur. Further investigations reveal that she has coarctation of the aorta. A karyotype was performed and the results were described as abnormal.

3) A 27-year-old woman attended for her routine anomaly ultrasound scan at 20 weeks' gestation. The fetus is found to have an echogenic focus in the heart and a nuchal fold of 8 mm. Amniocentesis was performed after counselling and the male fetus was found to have a balanced translocation.

4) A 30-year-old gravida 3 para 2 underwent an amniocentesis at 16 weeks' gestation because of balanced parental translocation. The male fetus is found to be carrying a robertsonian translocation.

5) During a routine ultrasound examination at 20 weeks' gestation, the fetus is found to have a strawberry head and is asymmetrically growth restricted. The liquor volume is normal but the uterine artery Dopplers show notches on both sides. An amniocentesis is performed and the female karyotype result is abnormal on FISH.

6) An amniocentesis is performed on a 24-year-old primigravida at 16 weeks because of a positive serum test. The karyotype shows that the fetus has a deletion on one of the long arms of a chromosome of the E group.

Option list for Questions 7–8

A.	Adhesiolysis
B.	Aromatase inhibitor – anastrozole
C.	Bilateral salpingo-oophorectomy
D.	Combined oral contraceptive pill
E.	Danazol
F.	Depo-Provera
G.	Drainage of ovarian endometrioma
H.	Gestodene
I.	GnRH agonist
J.	Laser ablation
K.	Levonorgestrel intrauterine system (Mirena)
L.	Medroxyprogesterone acetate (Provera)
M.	Mefenamic acid (Ponstan Forte)
N.	Ovarian cystectomy
O.	Total abdominal hysterectomy
P.	Total abdominal hysterectomy and bilateral salpingo-oophorectomy
Q.	Tranexamic acid (Cyklokapron)

Instructions: For each of the clinical scenarios described below, select from the option list above the **single** most suitable and effective first-line treatment that you will offer. Each option may be selected once, more than once or not at all.

7) A 32-year-old woman presents with heavy and painful periods of 3 years' duration. This started just before she had a multiload copper intrauterine device (IUD) inserted at the family planning clinic. She opted for the IUD as she did not think that she would remember to take her pills and her husband refused to be sterilized. On examination, she has mild bilateral adnexal tenderness but no other abnormality. A diagnostic laparoscopy revealed mild endometriosis in the pelvis.

8) A 20-year-old, single, slightly overweight woman, who is virgo intacta, presents with dysmenorrhoea and menorrhagia. Her periods are regular but have always been painful. Nothing is found on examination. At diagnostic laparoscopy, she is found to have mild endometriosis in the pelvis and ovaries.

Option list for Questions 9–11

A.	Cohort
B.	Cross-sectional
C.	Cross-sectional survey
D.	Dose–response
E.	Factorial design
F.	Longitudinal
G.	Matched control
H.	Mixed studies, randomized controlled
I.	Non-randomized historical controls
J.	Non-randomized prospective
K.	Pre-test/post-test
L.	Prospective cross-over
M.	Prospective non-randomized
N.	Prospective parallel
O.	Prospective randomized
P.	Randomized non-blinded
Q.	Randomized retrospective
R.	Retrospective deliberate intervention
S.	Retrospective observational
T.	Unmatched case control

Instructions: The following are details of various studies reported in various obstetrics and gynaecology journals over the last decade. Select from the above list the **single** option that best describes the study. Each option may be selected once, more than once or not at all.

9) Scott et al. (2008) conducted a trial of metformin or a placebo in women with gestational diabetes. After a 2-week run-in period, to allow the women to become familiar with the details of the trial, 40 volunteers were allocated by random selection either the metformin or the placebo tablets. After a month individual volunteers were crossed over to the alternative treatment for a further month. In the final week of each 1-month treatment period the percentage of glycated haemoglobin (HbA1c %) was measured.

10) A study was undertaken to determine the impact of education on the choice of contraceptive methods in a cohort of schoolgirls aged 16–17 years. Their methods of choice were first determined from a completed questionnaire, after which they were shown a video of various forms of contraception and the pros and cons of each. Another questionnaire was then administered and their chosen methods compared.

11) A team undertook a study of gonadotrophin levels in 18 women aged 35–42 years, 20 women aged 23–35 years presenting with menorrhagia and 20 healthy controls. The controls were healthy medical students.

Option list for Questions 12–14

A.	Combined oral contraceptive pill (COCP)
B.	Danazol
C.	Depo-Provera
D.	Dimetriose
E.	GnRH agonist
F.	Hysterectomy
G.	Levonorgestrel intrauterine system (Mirena)
H.	Mefenamic acid
I.	Myomectomy
J.	Norethisterone
K.	Polypectomy
L.	Thermal balloon endometrial ablation
M.	Tranexamic acid
N.	Transcervical resection of the endometrium
O.	Uterine fibroids

Instructions: For each of the following clinical scenarios, select the **single**, most appropriate, first-line treatment option from the above list. Each option may be chosen once, more than once or not at all.

12) A 30-year-old G2P2 presents with heavy and painful periods of 8 months' duration. The pains are spasmodic and associated with the passing of clots. Her husband had a vasectomy 3 years ago, after the birth of their second son. Her GP gave her tablets that she was taking only during menstruation, but they were not helping. Her mother had a similar problem and is currently suffering from

osteoporosis. On examination, her BMI is 22 kg/m^2 and the pelvic organs are essentially normal. Her Hb is 11.0 g/dL.

13) A 38-year-old G3P3 bank clerk presents with heavy and painful periods of 3 years' duration. She is fed up with this and reluctant to undergo any trial-and-error management as her GP has already put her through this for the past few years. On examination, her BMI is 26 kg/m^2 and her uterus is bulky. No obvious uterine fibroids are seen on the ultrasound scan, but the uterus is confirmed to be slightly enlarged. Her Hb is 10.3 g/dL.

14) A 39-year-old, severely hypertensive woman presents with heavy and painful periods of 12 months' duration. She also complains of severe premenstrual syndrome which has significantly affected the quality of her life. She is found, on examination, to have a BMI of 29 kg/m^2 and a normal size uterus. Her Hb is 10.4 g/dL.

Option list for Questions 15–19

A.	Admit for monitoring
B.	Change position and monitor CTG
C.	Continue with current management
D.	Discharge back to the community
E.	Emergency lower segment caesarean section (EMLSCS) under the third category (neither fetal nor maternal life threatening)
F.	Immediate caesarean section under general anaesthesia
G.	Immediate caesarean section under regional anaesthesia
H.	Instrumental delivery
I.	Monitor CTG for a further 5 minutes
J.	Monitor CTG for a further 30 minutes
K.	Repeat CTG
L.	Salbutamol – oral
M.	Stop Syntocinon
N.	Subcutaneous terbutaline
O.	Vaginal delivery as planned

Instructions: The following patients either presented to the delivery suite or are being managed on the delivery suite. For each case, select from the option list above the **single** most suitable immediate action plan. Each option may be selected once, more than once or not at all.

15) A primigravida was admitted to the labour ward at 4 cm dilatation. After 4 hours she was examined and found to be 8 cm dilated. She was contracting every minute and the CTG was showing reduced baseline variability and variable superficial deceleration. The liquor was blood stained. She has had an epidural.

16) A 40-year-old woman is admitted at 41 weeks with a free and mobile head. She is on a CTG which is showing decreased variability associated with variable decelerations.

17) A 38-year-old G2P1 admitted in labour at 40 weeks is found to have a CTG with decreased variability and late decelerations. Her cervix is 1 cm long and 1 cm dilated. Artificial rupture of fetal membranes revealed uniformly stained meconium liquor.

18) A senior house officer calls you for advice at 22 hours about a 40-year-old primigravida on the antenatal ward at 36 weeks' gestation who had been admitted because of unstable lie. The woman has been on a CTG for 20 minutes and it shows reduced variability and early decelerations.

19) A 34-year-old multiparous woman presents at term with a breech presentation. She is found to have multiple bruises over the abdomen. She had been kicked by her partner at home. A CTG was normal.

Option list for Questions 20–24

A.	Clomifene citrate
B.	Gonadotrophin therapy
C.	Danazol
D.	Estrogen-secreting tumour
E.	Herpes simplex virus type 2
F.	Human immunodeficiency virus (HIV)
G.	Human papillomavirus (HPV)
H.	Nulliparity
I.	Obesity
J.	Ovarian tumour
K.	Polycystic ovary syndrome
L.	Radiotherapy
M.	Talc powder
N.	Tamoxifen therapy
O.	Unopposed hormone replacement therapy

Instructions: The following clinical scenarios describe patients with various gynaecological malignancies. Choose from the option list above the **single** most likely aetiological factor of the malignancy. Each option may be chosen once, more than once or not at all.

20) A 45-year-old woman is diagnosed with an ovarian mass after presenting with a sudden-onset lower abdominal pain. She is nulliparous and had been treated unsuccessfully with tablets for infertility. At laparotomy she was found to have an ovarian cyst which was removed and sent for histology. It has come back as borderline serous cystadenoma.

21) A 29-year-old woman presented with postcoital bleeding and a brownish-red vaginal discharge of 4 months' duration. She has worked in the red light district of the city for the past 10 years and is being investigated for HIV. On examination, she is found to have an exophytic growth on the cervix suspicious of carcinoma.

22) A 43-year-old woman presented with irregular vaginal bleeding of 6 months' duration. She has three children and, as she was anovulatory, all were conceived after treatment with gonadotrophins. On examination her BMI is 30 kg/m^2. An endometrial biopsy has been reported as a well-differentiated carcinoma of the endometrium.

23) A 67 year old presents with postmenopausal bleeding of 2 months' durations. She had been receiving unopposed estrogen hormone replacement therapy until 10 years ago when it was stopped as she was found to have breast cancer. This was removed and she was placed on tamoxifen which she has been taking for 5 years. Her BMI is 28 kg/m^2. An endometrial biopsy has been reported as inflammation but there are focal areas of malignancy.

24) A 56-year-old woman presents with postmenopausal bleeding of 6 months' duration. She was found, on examination, to have a BMI of 26 kg/m^2, a normal size uterus for her age and an adnexal mass, which was confirmed on ultrasound scan to be an ovarian tumour. The endometrium was 9 mm thick and a biopsy has been reported as well-differentiated endometrial carcinoma.

Option list for Questions 25–26

A.	Anti-rho antibody
B.	Bronchoscopy for PCR
C.	CA-125
D.	Echocardiogram
E.	Chest X-ray
F.	C-reactive protein
G.	Computed tomography scan of the brain
H.	Electrocardiogram (ECG)
I.	Electroencephalogram (EEG)
J.	Fibrinogen degradation products
K.	Free thyroxine (FT_4)
L.	Four point blood glucose
M.	Glycated haemoglobin
N.	Oral glucose tolerance test
O.	Random blood glucose
P.	Renal ultrasound
Q.	Respiratory peak flow volume
R.	Thyroid-stimulating hormone
S.	24-hour ECG tape
T.	24-hour urinary protein
U.	Ultrasound scan – M-mode
V.	Urea and electrolytes

Instructions: For each of the following case scenarios described below, choose the **single** most useful confirmatory diagnostic test of the complication from the option list above. Each option may be chosen once, more than once or not at all.

25) A 29-year-old primigravida was referred by her midwife at 28 weeks' gestation with a BP of 160/110 mmHg. She booked for antenatal care at 16 weeks' gestation when her blood pressure was 150/95 mmHg. Her urine has remained clear of protein on dipstix throughout the pregnancy. Her Hb has remained low (highest 9.7 g/dL) throughout pregnancy, despite oral and parenteral iron supplementation. The peripheral film is suggestive of iron deficiency anaemia.

26) A 20-year-old, severely asthmatic woman presents at 16 weeks' gestation to the maternal medicine clinic. She is currently taking beta-sympathomimetics, which are thought to be controlling her asthma suboptimally. On examination, she is comfortable at rest although has mild rhonchi bilaterally.

Option list for Questions 27–30

A.	Advice against hormonal contraception
B.	Barrier method and estrogen vaginal cream
C.	Change combined oral contraceptive to IUD
D.	Combined HRT
E.	Continue combined contraceptives for 6 months and then stop if total duration of amenorrhoea since last spontaneous menses is at least 3 years
F.	Continue combined oral contraceptives for 12 months and then discontinue
G.	Continue combined oral contraceptives for 24 months and then stop
H.	Continue contraception for at least 2 years after the age of natural menopause
I.	Continuous combined HRT
J.	Continue contraception until blood tests confirm an ovulation
K.	Continue contraception until repeated blood tests show persistently raised FSH
L.	Continue with contraception for 1 year
M.	Discontinue contraception
N.	Endometrial biopsy and normal histology, start on the combined oral contraceptive
O.	Endometrial biopsy and start low-dose combined oral contraceptive pill if normal
P.	Measure FSH before discontinuing contraception
Q.	No need for contraception
R.	Progestogen-only contraceptive
S.	Raloxifene and continue with progestogen contraceptive
T.	Start on a low-dose combined oral contraceptive pill

Instructions: The women described below are in their perimenopausal years and have attended the routine gynaecology clinic for advice on contraception. For each patient select from the option list above the **single** most suitable advice that you would offer. Each option may be selected once, more than once or not at all.

27) A 51-year-old woman whose mother and sister attained menopause at the age of 48 years attends for contraceptive advice. She has been on the low-dose combined oral contraceptive pill for the past 5 years.

28) A 49-year-old woman presents with irregular periods. She is not currently on any form of contraception. Her last menstrual period was 3 weeks ago. Her BMI is 27 kg/m^2 and, on examination, nothing abnormal was been found.

29) A 52-year-old woman, whose last normal menstrual period was 1 year ago, wishes to go on the pill because her husband does not wish to continue using a condom. She is fit and well and there are no contraindications to the use of the combined oral contraceptive pill.

30) A 51-year-old woman who had a Mirena inserted 4 years ago has been amenorrhoeic for the past 3 years.

Option list for Questions 31–34

A.	Continue taking the pills but use a barrier method
B.	Discontinue contraception
C.	If the missed pill was after 7 days into the pack, take extra precautions and continue with the pills, missing out the forgotten one
D.	If the missed pill was 7 days into the pack, take the next pill and continue with the rest
E.	If the missed pill was 14 days into the pack, continue but take additional precautions for 7 days
F.	If the missed pill was 21 days into the pack, continue but take additional precautions until the next period
G.	If two pills are forgotten and these are within the first 7 days of the pack, take them immediately and continue the rest without additional precautions
H.	Stop the pills and avoid sexual intercourse
I.	Stop the pills and await the next period
J.	Stop the pills and await the next period but take additional precautions
K.	Take the forgotten pill and continue with the rest of the pack
L.	Take the forgotten pill(s) and use a barrier method until the next period
M.	Take the missed pill and continue with the remaining pills at the usual time.
N.	Take the missed pill and continue with the remaining pills at the usual time. Reassure about efficacy
O.	Take the missed pills now and the next pill as normal. No need to use additional contraception
P.	Take the missed pills now and the remaining one as normal; finish pack and skip the pill-free interval; start a new pack the next day and use additional contraception (condoms) for the next 7 days
Q.	Take the most recent pill now and continue taking the remaining pills daily at the usual time. Use condoms or abstain from sexual intercourse for 7 days. Emergency contraception should be offered
R.	Take the next pill and do a pregnancy test
S.	Take two pills and then continue with the rest of the pack

Instructions: The women described below presented after missing one or more oral contraceptive pills. They are concerned about an unplanned pregnancy and have sought your advice. For each patient, select from the above list of options the **single** most appropriate advice that you will offer. Each option may be selected once, more than once or not at all.

31) A 23-year-old female teacher has been on a low-dose (20 μg ethinyl-estradiol) combined oral contraceptive pill for the past 3 years. Unfortunately, she forgot to take two of her pills. She has four pills left in the pack.

32) An 18-year-old female student is taking Femodene ED (30 μg ethinyl-estradiol) but has missed two pills. She now has eight pills left in the packet.

33) A 22-year-old woman, who is on a 30 μg ethinylestradiol combined oral contraceptive pill, attends because she has missed three of her pills. She has only taken four pills in this pack and had unprotected sexual intercourse the night before.

34) A 37-year-old mother of three, who is on Cerazette (a progestogen-only contraceptive), attends because she had forgotten to take her pill 10 hours ago. She had sexual intercourse the night before.

A.	Stage 0 vagina carcinoma
B.	Stage I vaginal carcinoma
C.	Stage Ia vulval cancer
D.	Stage Ib vulval cancer
E.	Sage II vaginal carcinoma
F.	Stage II vulval cancer
G.	Stage III vaginal carcinoma
H.	Stage III vulval cancer
I.	Stage IVa vaginal carcinoma
J.	Stage IVa vulval cancer
K.	Stage IVb vaginal carcinoma
L.	Stage IVb vulval cancer
M.	VAIN (vaginal intraepithelial neoplasia) I
N.	VAIN II
O.	VAIN III
P.	VIN I
Q.	VIN II
R.	VIN III

Instructions: The following patients presented with symptoms of either vulval or vaginal malignancy. They were examined and ancillary investigations were undertaken prior to staging the disease. Select from the option list above the **single** most appropriate stage of the carcinoma. Each option may be selected once, more than once or not at all.

35) A 75-year-old woman presented with an ulcer on the vulva which was biopsied. This has been confirmed on histology to be carcinoma of the vulva confined to the vulva and with a maximum diameter of 1.5 cm.

36) An 82-year-old woman has just had an examination under anaesthesia and a biopsy of a suspicious lesion of the vulva. The lesion, which was confined to the left labium majorum, measured 3.5 cm. There were no palpable groin nodes. This has now been confirmed to be squamous carcinoma of the vulva.

37) A 78-year-old woman presents with a mass on the vulva which extends into the lower vagina. She has bilaterally enlarged groin nodes. A biopsy of the mass has confirmed it to be carcinoma of the vulva.

38) An 80-year-old woman presented with postmenopausal bleeding and was found, on examination, to have a lesion on the upper third of the vagina. This was biopsied and histology confirmed it to be carcinoma of the vagina confined to the epithelium.

39) A 77-year-old frail woman presented with rectal bleeding which was described by the GP as secondary to haemorrhoids. At examination under anaesthesia, this was found to be a mass that also involved the vagina. A biopsy was obtained and this has been shown to be carcinoma of the vagina.

40) A 60-year-old woman had a routine cervical smear which was reported as suspicious. She had a colposcopy and some suspicious areas were identified in the vagina. The cervix was, however, normal. A biopsy of one of these lesions has been reported as carcinoma with no subepithelial tissue involvement.

8. Practice Paper 8: Answers

Note: These questions are quite straightforward if candidates have a good understanding of the arrangement and structure of chromosomes.

1) **Q.**
Patau's syndrome is a trisomy. All the answers that are not trisomies can easily be eliminated if the candidate knows what trisomies are. The correct answer is trisomy 13.

2) **A.**
The clinical features described are those of Turner's syndrome which is 45 XO.

3) **P.**
There are two balanced translocations in the list of options. One is female and the other is male. This makes identifying the correct answer easy.

4) **D.**
There are two options with robertsonian translocations – one is male and the other is female.

5) **R.**
The clinical features are those of Edward's syndrome which is trisomy 18.

6) **H.**
Human chromosomes are grouped into seven groups. Group A are chromosomes 1–3, group B chromosomes 4–5, group C chromosomes 6–12 and X, group D chromosomes 13–15, group E chromosomes 16–18, group F chromosomes 19–20 and group G chromosomes 21–22 and Y.

7) **K.**
An ideal treatment of this patient's endometriosis will be one that does not require her to remember to take her medication. The best option is, therefore, the levonorgestrel intrauterine system.

8) **L.**
Progestogens are an effective treatment of the symptoms of endometriosis. In an obese patient, the 17-C or less androgenic progestogens should be offered. As Duphaston has been discontinued, the best option would be Provera.

9) L.

This is a prospective cross-over test as explained in the question. After I month the groups were crossed over to the alternative treatment.

10) K.

This is a pre-test–post-test study.

11) T.

This is an unmatched study as the groups were not matched for any specific parameters, including age.

12) A.

A variety of options is available to this patient, including dimetriose, GnRH agonists, the Mirena and the combined oral contraceptive pill. With a family history of osteoporosis, a GnRH agonist should be considered only after she has had bone densitometry to exclude osteopenia. A similar caution would be exercised with the use of dimetriose. The COCP would be an ideal option, although the Mirena could be used as a second option.

13) F.

As the patient has tried different medications with no success, and because she is 38 years old and has three children, a hysterectomy would be the best option.

14) E.

Although surgery and the Mirena are options for this obese patient, they are both associated with side effects. If her ovaries are not taken out, she will continue to suffer the severe premenstrual syndrome. The best option would, therefore, be to suppress the ovarian activity with a GnRH agonist.

15) F.

This patient is having hypertonic uterine contractions and, as she is not on Syntocinon, the blood-stained amniotic fluid will suggest an abruption. The baby requires an emergency delivery. Since she has had an epidural, this should be done under a regional anaesthetic.

16) B.

The woman has an unstable lie and, therefore, the abnormality seen on the CTG may be related to cord compression. Her position should be changed and the CTG continued before any decisions on further action are taken.

17) E.

This baby needs to be delivered but there are no fetal or maternal life-threatening indications.

18) **B**.

The admission was for an unstable lie and the CTG has been recorded for only 20 minutes. The position of the patient should be changed and the CTG continued.

19) **A**.

The risks to this woman include further physical injury by the partner. However, delayed-onset placental abruption cannot be excluded and, therefore, it is essential to admit her, not only in order to monitor the baby but to remove her from immediate danger.

20) **A**.

Borderline ovarian tumours are not uncommonly associated with infertility treatments, especially clomifene induction of ovulation.

21) **G**.

Carcinoma of the cervix is considered a sexually transmitted infection. In more than 70% of cases, HPV infection is the underlying cause. This is very likely to be the case for this patient.

22) **K**.

Endometrial carcinoma is rare in those younger than 40 years. When it does occur, in this age group and in those in their 40s, there is most likely to be higher circulating estrogen levels as seen in PCOS.

23) **N**.

Tamoxifen is an anti-estrogen with selective estrogenic action on the endometrium. Its use is associated with the development of endometrial cancer. This is common after at least 5 years of treatment.

24) **D**.

Postmenopausal bleeding and an adnexal mass are highly indicative of an estrogen-secreting ovarian tumour.

25) **P**.

This patient is hypertensive and has iron deficiency anaemia that is not responding to iron supplementation. This will suggest a renal cause of the anaemia and an ultrasound scan will be a useful investigation.

26) **Q**.

The patient requires an assessment of her lung functions and the best option is a respiratory peak flow measurement. There is no evidence that she has an infection and a chest X-ray will not provide any useful information. An ECG and echocardiogram will not be useful.

27) M.

The patient does not require any further contraception. She is most likely to have attained menopause as her sister and mother attained menopause at the age of 48 years. The natural age at menopause in the UK is 51–52 years.

28) O.

It is important to establish that she does not have any endometrial pathology before contraception can be offered. A biopsy should, therefore, be performed and, if it is normal, the combined oral contraceptive pill would be suitable as it will also regularize her periods.

29) Q.

The patient does not need contraception as she is postmenopausal.

30) L.

This patient should continue with the Mirena for at least 12 months before having it removed.

31) P.

The patient should take the missed pills now and the remaining one as normal. She should finish the pack, skip the pill-free interval and start a new pack the next day. She should also use an additional contraception (condom) for the next 7 days.

32) O.

The patient should take the missed pills now and the next pill as normal. There is no need for her to use additional contraception.

33) Q.

The patient should take the most recent pill now and continue taking the remaining pills daily at the usual time. She should also use condoms, or abstain from sexual intercourse, for 7 days. Emergency contraception should be offered to her.

34) M.

She should be advised to take the missed pill and continue with the remaining pills at the usual time. The safety window with Cerazette is 12 hours compared with 3 hours with other progestogen-only pills.

Note: These questions are straightforward and the answers are simply the most appropriate stage of vulval or vaginal carcinoma.

35) C.
Stage Ia carcinoma of the vulva.

36) F.
Stage II carcinoma of the vulva.

37) H.
Stage III carcinoma of the vulva.

38) B.
Stage I carcinoma of the vagina.

39) I.
Stage IVa carcinoma of the vagina.

40) B.
Stage I carcinoma of the vagina.